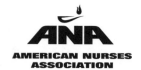

AMERICAN NURSES ASSOCIATION

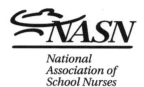

National
Association of
School Nurses

Scope AND
Standards
OF PRACTICE

School
Nursing

2ND EDITION

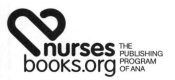

nurses
books.org THE
PUBLISHING
PROGRAM
OF ANA

American Nurses Association
Silver Spring, Maryland
2011

Library of Congress Cataloging-in-Publication Data

School nursing : scope and standards of practice. — 2nd ed.
    p. ; cm.
  Includes bibliographical references and index.
    Summary: "Describes and delineates the expectations and parameters of the professional
role of the U.S. school nurse across all practice settings by detailing the activities, accountabilities,
competencies - the expected professional performance levels that integrate knowledge, skills, abilities,
and judgment - education and professional development, and other key school nursing traits and
qualifications"—Provided by publisher.
    ISBN-13: 978-1-55810-353-5 (pbk. : alk. paper)
    ISBN-10: 1-55810-353-8 (pbk. : alk. paper)
    ISBN-13: 978-1-55810-352-8 (eBook, PDF format)
    ISBN-13: 978-1-55810-354-2 (eBook, EPUB format)
    ISBN-13: 978-1-55810-355-9 (eBook, Mobipocket format)

  1. School nursing—Standards—United States. I. National Association of School Nurses (U.S.)
  II. American Nurses Association. [DNLM: 1. School Nursing—Practice Guideline. 2. School Health
      Services—Practice Guideline.   WY 113]
  RJ247.N38 2011
  371.7'12—dc23
                                                                                            2011017470

The American Nurses Association (ANA) is a national professional association. This ANA publication—
School Nursing: Scope and Standards of Practice, Second Edition—reflects the thinking of the nursing
profession on various issues related to school nursing and should be reviewed in conjunction with
state board of nursing policies and practices. State law, rules, and regulations govern the practice
of nursing, while *School Nursing: Scope and Standards of Practice, Second Edition,* guides nurses in
the application of their professional skills and responsibilities. For more about the American Nurses
Association and the National Association of School Nurses, see pages ix and x. The information in this
book should not be construed or interpreted as legal or professional advice.

Published by Nursesbooks.org
The Publishing Program of ANA
www.Nursesbooks.org/

American Nurses Association
8515 Georgia Avenue, Suite 400
Silver Spring, MD 20910-3492
1-800-274-4ANA
www.NursingWorld.org

    ISBN-13: 978-1-55810-353-5   SAN: 851-3481   2K   10/2014R

    First printing: July, 2011. Second printing: September, 2013. Third printing: October 2014

Contents

Contributors

NASN Work Group Members

Elizabeth L. Thomas, MEd, BS, RN, NCSN, FNASN (Chair), Delaware
Editor and Standards Task Force Leader, *School Nursing: Scope and Standards of Practice* (2005); Past Board and Executive Board Member, National Association of School Nurses; Past President, Delaware School Nurse Association; School Nurse and School Nurse Coordinator (retired), Christina School District, Wilmington, Delaware; Consultant, *School Health Consulting*, Wilmington, Delaware.

Julia Muennich Cowell, PhD, APHN-BC, FAAN, Illinois
Executive Editor, *The Journal of School Nursing*; Member, Standards Task Force, 2005; Professor Emerita, College of Nursing, Rush University, Chicago, Illinois.

Linda Davis-Alldritt, MA, RN, PHN, FNASN, FASHA, California
President-Elect, National Association of School Nurses; Past President of National Association of State School Nurse Consultants; State School Nurse Consultant, California Department of Education; Member, Standards Task Force, 2005; Past President, California School Nurses Organization.

Sandra Delack, MEd, BSN, RN, NCSN, Rhode Island
President, National Association of School Nurses; Health Services Coordinator, Johnston Public Schools, Johnston, Rhode Island; and School Nurse-Teacher, N.A. Ferri Middle School, Johnston, Rhode Island.

Janice Doyle, MSN, RN, NCSN, FNASN, Washington
Past Board and Executive Board Member, National Association of School Nurses; Lead School Nurse, Bethel School District, Spanaway, Washington; Clinical Affiliate Faculty, Pacific Lutheran University, Tacoma, Washington.

Beverly Hine, MPH, RN, NCSN, FASHA, New Mexico
Board and Executive Board Member, National Association of School Nurses; Director, Health Services/Medicaid, Las Cruces Public Schools, Las Cruces, New Mexico.

Donna Mazyck, MS, RN, NCSN, Maryland
Past President, National Association of School Nurses; State School Nurse Consultant, Maryland State Department of Education, Baltimore, Maryland.

Kathleen Patrick, MA, RN, NCSN, FNASN, Colorado
Past Board and Nominating Committee Member, National Association of School Nurses; Director-at-Large, National Association of State School Nurses Consultants; Assistant Director, Health and Wellness Unit, State School Nurse Consultant, Colorado Department of Education, Denver, Colorado.

Susan E. Proctor, DNS, MPH, RN, FNASN, California
Author, "Standards of Practice: What They Are and How to Use Them" (in Selekman [Ed.], 2006, 2012); Member, NASN Standards Task Force, 1998; Author, *School Nursing: Roles and Standards*, NASN, 1993; Past Executive Editor, *The Journal of School Nursing*, 1996–1999; Author, *To See or Not to See: Screening the Vision of Children in School*, NASN, 2005; Professor Emerita, School of Nursing, California State University, Sacramento, California.

Cheryl Resha, EdD, MSN, RN, Connecticut
Immediate past NASN Representative on the American Nurses Association Congress on Nursing Practice and Economics; Past President of National Association of State School Nurse Consultants; State Director of Child Nutrition and School Health Programs, Connecticut State Department of Education, Middletown, Connecticut.

Linda C. Wolfe, MEd, BSN, RN, NCSN, FNASN, Delaware
NASN Representative on the American Nurses Association Congress on Nursing Practice and Economics; Past President of National Association of School Nurses; State School Nurse Consultant and Director, School Support Services, Delaware Department of Education, Delaware; Member, NASN Standards Task Force, 1998.

Consultant on Healthy School Environment

Norma Bergey, MSN, RN, NCSN, Virginia
President, Virginia Association of School Nurses; School Nurse at G.W. Carver Intermediate School, Chesapeake, Virginia; Consultant to Task Force regarding healthy school environment.

Resources

The work group wishes to acknowledge the work on school nurse competencies done by school nurses and others in Connecticut and New Mexico (Connecticut State Department of Education [CSDE], 2009; New Mexico Public Education Department [NMPED], 2006). Some competencies were derived from prior standards work sponsored by the National Association of School Nurses and the American Nurses Association (Appendix A). In addition, *Public Health Nursing: Scope and Standards of Practice* (ANA, 2007b) served as a valued resource.

ANA Staff

Carol J. Bickford, PhD, RN-BC, CPHIMS – Content editor
Yvonne Daley Humes, MSA – Project coordinator
Maureen E. Cones, Esq. – Legal counsel
Eric Wurzbacher – Project editor
Melaney Johnson – Printing and manufacturing coordinator

About the National Association of School Nurses

The National Association of School Nurses (NASN) is a nonprofit specialty nursing organization, organized in 1968 and incorporated in 1977, representing school nurses exclusively. NASN has over 15,000 members and 51 affiliates, including in the District of Columbia and overseas. The mission of the NASN is "to improve the health and educational success of children and youth by developing and providing leadership to advance the school nursing practice." More at http://www.nasn.org/

About the American Nurses Association

The American Nurses Association (ANA) is the only full-service professional organization representing the interests of the nation's 3.1 million registered nurses through its constituent/state nurses associations and its organizational affiliates. The ANA advances the nursing profession by fostering high standards of nursing practice, promoting the rights of nurses in the workplace, projecting a positive and realistic view of nursing, and lobbying the Congress and regulatory agencies on healthcare issues affecting nurses and the public. More at www.NursingWorld.org

About Nursesbooks.org, the Publishing Program of ANA

Nursesbooks.org publishes books on ANA core issues and programs, including ethics, leadership, quality, specialty practice, advanced practice, and the profession's enduring legacy. Best known for the foundational documents of the profession on ethics, scope and standards of practice, and social policy, Nursesbooks.org is the publisher for the professional, career-oriented nurse, reaching and serving nurse educators, administrators, managers, and researchers, as well as staff nurses during the course of their professional development. More at www.Nursesbooks.org/

Preface

Standards have a practical, not just formal value. Within school nursing, standards are professional expectations that guide the practice of school nursing. As such, they are valuable allies for the school nurse in developing position descriptions, crafting performance appraisal instruments, evaluating the quality of the school health program, communicating with non-nurse school administrators, and describing the role of the nurse in legal proceedings. Finally, and perhaps most important, standards reaffirm for the school nurse the essence of school nursing and the scope of school nursing practice (adapted from Proctor, in press).

Setting the Stage

Relationship of School Nursing's Foundational Documents

School Nursing: Scope and Standards of Practice, Second Edition, describes and measures a competent level of school nursing practice and professional performance. Registered nurses practicing in the United States as school nurses have some key professional resources that inform their thinking and decision-making and guide their practice. First, *Code of Ethics for Nurses with Interpretive Statements* (ANA, 2001), *Guide to the Code of Ethics for Nurses: Interpretation and Application* (Fowler, 2008), and *Code of Ethics with Interpretive Statements for the School Nurse* (NASN, 2010b) list the succinct provisions that establish the ethical framework for registered nurses and school nurses across all roles, levels, and settings. Second, *Nursing's Social Policy Statement: The Essence of the Profession* (ANA, 2010b) conceptualizes nursing practice, describes the social context of nursing, and provides the definition of nursing. The third resource is *Nursing: Scope and Standards of Practice, Second Edition* (ANA, 2010a). This foundational document outlines the expectations of the professional role of the registered nurse and presents the Standards of Professional Nursing Practice for all registered nurses with accompanying competencies. It is this document on which the scope and standards of school nursing practice are based.

Audience

School nurses, school nurse administrators, and registered nurses constitute the primary audience of this professional resource. Healthcare providers, healthcare systems, agencies and organizations, school district administrators, school board members, and interprofessional colleagues also will find this a valuable reference in understanding the role of school nurses, the supervision of nursing personnel and unlicensed assistive personnel (UAP) in schools, and the development of the school health program. In addition, students, families, communities, and other populations using nursing services in the school and health care in the community can use this document to better understand what comprises the practice of school nursing and who its members are: registered nurses, advanced practice registered nurses, and graduate-level prepared school nurses. Finally, legislators, regulators, legal counsel, and the judiciary system may wish to reference this document, describing the scope of school nursing practice and the accompanying specialty standards of practice and professional performance.

Scope of School Nursing Practice

Definitions and Distinguishing Characteristics of School Nursing Practice

Definitions

"Nursing is the protection, promotion, and optimization of health and abilities, prevention of illness and injury, alleviation of suffering through the diagnosis and treatment of human response, and advocacy in the care of individuals, families, communities, and populations" (ANA, 2010a, p. 1; ANA, 2010b, p. 10).

"School nursing is a specialized practice of professional nursing that advances the well-being, academic success, and life-long achievement and health of students. To that end, school nurses facilitate positive student responses to normal development; promote health and safety, including a healthy environment; intervene with actual and potential health problems; provide case management services; and actively collaborate with others to build student and family capacity for adaptation, self-management, self-advocacy, and learning" (NASN, 2010c).

Distinguishing Characteristics

The American Nurses Association identifies the following attributes that "truly reflect the definition of nursing and illustrate the *essential features of contemporary nursing practice*" [italics added]:

- A caring relationship that facilitates health and healing

- Attention to a range of human experiences and responses to health, disease, and illness in the physical and social environments

- Integration of objective data with knowledge gained from an appreciation of the healthcare consumer's or group's subjective experience

- Application of scientific knowledge to diagnosis and treatment through the use of judgment and critical thinking

- Advancement of professional nursing knowledge through scholarly inquiry

- Influence on social and public policy to promote social justice

- Assurance of safe, quality, and evidence-based practice

(ANA, 2010a, pp. 28–29; ANA, 2010b, p. 9).

School Nursing's Scope and Standards of Practice

Description of the Scope of School Nursing Practice

The scope of practice statement describes the "who," "what," "where," "when," "why," and "how" of school nursing practice. Each of these questions must be sufficiently answered to provide a complete picture of the dynamic and complex practice of school nursing and its evolving boundaries and membership. The specialty of school nursing has one scope of practice that encompasses a broad range of nursing practice. The depth and breadth in which individual school nurses engage in the total scope of school nursing practice depend on education, experience, role, work environment, and the population served.

Function of School Nursing Standards

The standards of school nursing practice are authoritative statements of the duties that school nurses, regardless of role, population, or specialty within school nursing, are expected to competently perform (adapted from ANA, 2010a, p. 2). The standards published herein may be utilized as evidence of a legal standard of care and govern school nurses practicing within the role, population, and specialty governed by this document. The standards are subject to change: with the dynamics of the school nursing specialty; as new patterns of professional practice are developed and accepted by school nursing, the education community, and the public; as new expectations for the academic success and life-long achievement of students are articulated; and as changes in societal trends occur. "Standards are subject to formal, periodic review and revision" (ANA, 2010a, p. 31).

This document includes 21 standards statements that, by themselves, serve the nurse and schools as a framework for outlining an expansive scope of practice. The language is intentionally broad and serves to paint an overall picture of practice. The standards statements become more effective, however, as a comprehensive and refined listing of expectations essential to practice without further development and explication. Furthermore, "the roles and activities in which the school nurse engages, particularly as the nurse uses the nursing process, may be state and/or district specific, and the uniqueness of a given position cannot be fully understood, comprehended, or appreciated through the use of standards statements by themselves. Standards statements, therefore, optimally serve nursing practice or the recipients of nursing care when further tailored to the specifics of the focus or setting" (Proctor, in press).

Each standards statement is accompanied by several basic competencies. The competency statements in turn may be further specified as befits the practice setting. Proctor (in press) has further described competencies as specific, measurable elements that interpret, explain, and facilitate practical use of a standard. The competencies may be evidence of compliance with the individual standard but are not exhaustive and depend on the circumstances. Competencies may be used by school nursing professionals to appraise professional performance and for other purposes. School nurses can identify opportunities for development and improvement of their practice by evaluating personal performance based on these competency statements. School nurses can also use the competencies to inform school administrators and others as to practice expectations.

In school nursing, the practice context must be considered in the use of standards. A registered nurse employed full time in special education, for example, responsible for the care of children with severe disabilities, will and should be evaluated somewhat differently than the nurse in regular education. In addition, specific conditions and practice circumstances may also affect the application of the standards and their accompanying competencies, for example, student ratio and acuity, a natural disaster or school lockdown, and character of the work environment.

Origin of School Nursing Standards

Professional nursing and nursing specialty organizations have a responsibility to their members and to the public they serve to develop standards of practice. As the professional organization for all registered nurses, the American

Nurses Association (ANA) has assumed the responsibility for developing standards that apply to the practice of all registered nurses and serve as a template for the development of school nursing standards as specialty standards. "Standards . . . belong to the profession and, thus, require broad input into their development and revision" (ANA, 2010a, pp. 1–2).

History of School Nursing Standards

Standards of professional school nursing practice pertain to the specialty practice of school nursing. Throughout the early and mid-20th century, many school nurses and professional nursing groups attempted to define school nursing and articulate roles and functions, both essential to the development of standards (Appendix A). Others outside of nursing also weighed in. Reflective of the considerable paternalism of the day, a joint committee of the National Education Association and the American Medical Association authored a paper titled, *The Nurse in the School*, that defined and laid down a role for nursing in schools (Joint Committee, 1941).

By 1960, no fewer than five groups were speaking for school nursing with the School Nurses Branch, Public Health Nursing Section of the ANA, and the Committee on School Nursing Policies and Practices of the American School Health Association, representing the majority of school nurses. These groups authored significant papers on the role and function of school nursing (Appendix A). By 1970, the Department of School Nurses of the National Education Association (NEA), later to become the National Association of School Nurses (NASN), had grown in influence among school nurses and published a role and function paper of its own (NEA Department of School Nurses, 1970).

In 1983, after eight decades of identifying and refining the role of the school nurse, the first national standards of practice were developed when several organizations, all interested in school nursing, came together under the leadership and direction of the NASN to produce a set of standards modeled on a template laid down by the ANA (ANA, 1983). The current document, *School Nursing: Scope and Standards of Practice, Second Edition*, is the latest of several sets of published school nursing standards using an ANA-stipulated format and describes a competent level of nursing practice and professional performance common to and expected of all school nurses.

Tenets of School Nursing Practice

Five tenets characterize contemporary school nursing practice:

1. Nursing practice is individualized.

School nursing practice is respectful of diversity and is individualized to meet the unique needs of the healthcare consumer in or associated with the school environment. The healthcare consumer in the school community is defined as the individual, family, group, community, or population who is the focus of attention and to whom the school nurse is providing services as sanctioned by the state regulatory bodies.

2. Nurses coordinate care by establishing partnerships.

The school nurse establishes partnerships with persons, families, communities, support systems, and other providers, utilizing in-person and electronic communication methods, to reach a shared goal of delivering health care. *Health care* is defined as the attempt "to address the health needs of the patient and the public" (ANA, 2001, p. 10). Collaborative, interprofessional team planning is based on recognition of each discipline's value and contributions, mutual trust, respect, open discussion, and shared decision-making. The school nurse coordinates with the student's healthcare home to better serve the healthcare consumer.

3. Caring is central to the practice of the school nurse.

Professional school nursing promotes healing and health in a way that builds a relationship between school nurse and healthcare consumers (adapted from Watson, 1999, 2008). "Caring is a conscious judgment that manifests itself in concrete acts, interpersonally, verbally, and non-verbally" (Gallagher-Lepak & Kubsch, 2009, p. 171). While caring for individuals, families, and populations is the key focus of school nursing, the school nurse additionally promotes self-care, as well as care of the environment and society (Hagerty, Lynch-Sauer, Patusky, & Bouwsema, 1993).

4. Registered nurses use the nursing process to plan and provide individualized care to their patients.

School nurses use theoretical and evidence-based knowledge of human experiences and responses to advocate for and collaborate with healthcare consumers in assessing, diagnosing, identifying outcomes, planning, implementing, and evaluating care. Nursing interventions are intended to produce beneficial effects, contribute to quality outcomes, and above all, do no harm. "Nurses evaluate the effectiveness of their care in relation to identified outcomes and use evidence-based practice to improve care" (ANA, 2010a, pp. 4–5). Critical thinking underlies each step of the nursing, problem-solving, and decision-making processes. The nursing process is often conceptualized and presented as the integration of the *singular* concurrent actions of assessment, diagnosis, identification of outcomes, planning, implementation, and evaluation (adapted from ANA, 2010b, p. 22). In practice, the nursing process is not linear but continuous and circular, with each step informing both the previous step and the succeeding step. The nursing process, then, is cyclical and dynamic, client centered, interpersonal and collaborative, and universally applicable. Furthermore, in many school nursing situations, the process is ongoing and long term (ANA, 2010a, p. 5; Proctor, in press).

5. A strong link exists between the professional work environment and the registered nurse's ability to provide quality patient care and achieve optimal patient outcomes.

Professional school nurses have an ethical obligation to maintain and improve healthcare environments conducive to the provision of quality health care (ANA, 2001). Elements of a healthy work environment have been extensively studied and document the relationship between effective practice and quality of the work environment. The school nurse must maintain and improve the healthcare environment for both the nurse and healthcare consumers.

Healthy Work Environments for School Nursing

Evidence demonstrates that negative, demoralizing, and unsafe conditions in the workplace, emanating from a physically or psychologically unhealthy environment, contribute to nursing errors, ineffective delivery of care, and conflict and stress among health or other professionals and those they serve. The school nurse is expected to contribute toward the reduction or elimination of physical and psychological health risks in the school setting.

The Institute of Medicine (IOM, 2004) has reported that safety and quality problems exist when dedicated health professionals work within systems that neither prepare nor support them in achieving optimal client care outcomes.

Rapid changes, such as reimbursement modification and cost-containment efforts, new healthcare technologies, and changes in the healthcare workforce, have influenced the work and work environment of all nurses. Concentration on key aspects of the work environment, encompassing people, physical places, and tools, can enhance healthcare working conditions and improve safety. These include transformational leadership and evidence-based management; maximizing workforce capability; creating and sustaining a culture of safety and research; work space design and redesign to prevent and mitigate errors; addressing potential pollutants in the work environment; and the effective use of telecommunications.

The establishment and maintenance of a healthy work environment require all nurses to (1) be proficient in skilled communication; (2) foster true collaboration with partners; (3) be effective decision-makers in policy and in leading organizations; (4) ensure appropriate staffing; (5) foster recognition of self and others; and (6) embrace the role of a leader in creating and sustaining a healthy work environment (AACN, 2005). These principles of a healthy employment environment apply aptly to school nurses who must work as health professionals in an education environment. This requires the school nurse to collaborate often and well; to communicate the important contributions of nursing to academic success with those in the education field; and to assume leadership roles in student assistance teams, wellness committees, and staff health promotion policies and activities.

Ratios and Caseloads

Work-related environmental issues particularly relevant to school nurses are ratios and caseloads. Many times, caseloads assigned to individual school nurses are unrealistic and unmanageable. For health and safety reasons, implementing reasonable ratios is essential.

NASN recommends the following minimum ratios of school nurses to students, depending on the needs of the student populations: 1:750 for students in the general population; 1:225 in student populations that may require daily professional school nursing services or interventions; 1:125 in student populations with complex healthcare needs; and 1:1 as necessary for individual students who require daily and continuous professional nursing services (Garcia, 2009, p. 198).

In rural areas, the recommended ratio may not be appropriate if geographic distance between schools is such that nurses spend inordinate time traveling, even if the ratio meets NASN recommendations. Caseload must always be a consideration in the promotion of a healthy work environment and should be based on the needs of clients. Increased need for nursing care and intervention requires an adaptable caseload to meet student healthcare management needs and to facilitate the delivery of health promotion programs (NASN, 2010a).

Environmental Health Considerations

The environmental component of the Coordinated School Health Program (CSHP) provides a model for a physically and psychologically healthy work and learning environment and suggests that the school nurse monitor, report, and intervene as necessary to promote and support a healthy environment (Allensworth & Kolbe as cited in Marx, Wooley, & Northrop, 1998; CDC, 2010a; Thomas, 2006). (The CSHP is central to a national strategy for improving health and learning in schools. The mission of academic success of students and staff is strongly linked to the health of students, staff, families, and community. For details, see pages 22 and 23.)

Such ongoing efforts continue some of the earliest aspects of school nursing. Pioneering public health nurses Lillian Wald (who was also an early leader in school nursing) and Florence Nightingale demonstrated that cleanliness in the environment affected the health of their patients and suggested that all nurses practice cleanliness (Nightingale, 1860/1969; Wolfe, in press). In 2010, the United States Environmental Protection Agency (U.S. EPA, 2010a) reported that more than 53 million children and 6 million adults spend school days in more than 120,000 private and public schools. The report suggested that the age and condition of school buildings, as well as inconsistent opportunities for hand washing, may affect health and the ability to learn and teach (U.S. EPA, 2010b). The NASN states that school nurses are in a position to advocate for a "safe school environment because of their close contact with staff, students, families, community members, and healthcare providers" (NASN, 2005).

Today's school environment can be filled with many types of environmental toxins and communicable and infectious agents that can affect the health and welfare of students and others in the school community. The school nurse, as the health expert in the school, can help to mitigate or eliminate environmental pollutants and pathogenic organisms in the school setting. Finally, the school nurse contributes to safeguarding the environment by participating in the development and implementation of emergency and disaster preparedness plans.

Overview of the Standards of School Nursing Practice

The Standards of School Nursing Practice consist of Standards of Practice and Standards of Professional Performance. The Standards of Practice are the six steps of the nursing process. The use of the nursing process as standards represents the directive nature of the standards as the school nurse completes each component of the nursing process. Similarly, the standards of professional performance relate to how the school nurse adheres to all the standards of practice and addresses other nursing practice issues, concerns, and activities. See Figure 1.

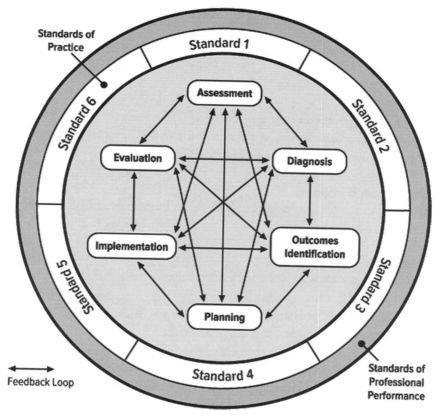

FIGURE 1. Nursing Process and Standards of Professional Nursing Practice
Source: ANA 2010a, p. 3.

Standards of Practice for School Nursing

The Standards of Practice for School Nursing describe a competent level of nursing care as demonstrated by the critical thinking model known as the nursing process. The nursing process includes the components of assessment, diagnosis, outcomes identification, planning, implementation, and evaluation. These standards encompass all significant actions taken by registered nurses and form the foundation of the school nurse's decision-making (adapted from ANA, 2010a, p. 9; ANA, 2010b, p. 22).

The Standards of Practice for School Nursing are as follows:

STANDARD 1. ASSESSMENT

The school nurse collects comprehensive data pertinent to the healthcare consumer's health and/or the situation.

STANDARD 2. DIAGNOSIS

The school nurse analyzes the assessment data to determine the diagnoses or issues.

STANDARD 3. OUTCOMES IDENTIFICATION

The school nurse identifies expected outcomes for a plan individualized to the healthcare consumer or the situation.

STANDARD 4. PLANNING

The school nurse develops a plan that prescribes strategies and alternatives to attain expected outcomes.

STANDARD 5. IMPLEMENTATION

The school nurse implements the identified plan.

STANDARD 5A. COORDINATION OF CARE

The school nurse coordinates care delivery.

STANDARD 5B. HEALTH TEACHING AND HEALTH PROMOTION

The school nurse uses strategies to promote a healthy and a safe environment, especially regarding health education.

STANDARD 5C. CONSULTATION

The school nurse provides consultation to influence the identified plan, enhance the abilities of others, and effect change.

STANDARD 5D. PRESCRIPTIVE AUTHORITY AND TREATMENT
The advanced practice registered nurse uses prescriptive authority, procedures, referrals, treatments, and therapies in accordance with state and federal laws and regulations.

STANDARD 6. EVALUATION
The school nurse evaluates progress toward attainment of outcomes.

Standards of Professional Performance for School Nursing

The Standards of Professional Performance for School Nursing describe a competent level of behavior in the professional role. Areas of expected professional performance include ethics, education, evidence-based practice and research, quality of practice, communication, leadership, collaboration, professional practice evaluation, resource utilization, environmental health, and program management. All school nurses are expected to actively engage in professional role activities appropriate to their education and position. School nurses are accountable for their professional actions to themselves, their healthcare consumers, the profession, and, ultimately, to society (adapted from ANA, 2010a, p. 10; ANA, 2010b, p. 22).

The Standards of Professional Performance for School Nursing are as follows:

STANDARD 7. ETHICS
The school nurse practices ethically.

STANDARD 8. EDUCATION
The school nurse attains knowledge and competency that reflect current nursing practice.

STANDARD 9. EVIDENCE-BASED PRACTICE AND RESEARCH
The school nurse integrates evidence and research findings into practice.

STANDARD 10. QUALITY OF PRACTICE
The school nurse contributes to quality nursing practice.

STANDARD 11. COMMUNICATION
The school nurse communicates effectively in a variety of formats in all areas of nursing practice.

STANDARD 12. LEADERSHIP
The school nurse demonstrates leadership in the professional practice setting and the profession.

STANDARD 13. COLLABORATION
The school nurse collaborates with the healthcare consumer, family, and others in the conduct of nursing practice.

STANDARD 14. PROFESSIONAL PRACTICE EVALUATION
The school nurse evaluates one's own nursing practice in relation to professional practice standards and guidelines, relevant statutes, rules, and regulations.

STANDARD 15. RESOURCE UTILIZATION
The school nurse utilizes appropriate resources to plan and provide nursing services that are safe, effective, and financially responsible.

STANDARD 16. ENVIRONMENTAL HEALTH
The school nurse practices in an environmentally safe and healthy manner.

STANDARD 17. PROGRAM MANAGEMENT
The school nurse manages school health services.

Competence and Competency in School Nursing Practice

The school community has a right to expect school nurses to demonstrate professional competence throughout their careers. The school nurse is individually responsible and accountable for maintaining professional competence. Beyond individual responsibility, the NASN and the ANA further believe that it is the nursing profession's responsibility to shape and guide any process for assuring nurse competence. Regulatory agencies define minimal standards for regulation of nursing practice to protect the public. Finally, the employer is responsible and accountable for providing and accountable for an environment conducive to competent school nursing practice. Therefore, assurance of competence is the shared responsibility of the profession, individual school nurses, professional organizations, credentialing and certification entities, regulatory agencies, employers, and other key stakeholders (adapted from ANA, 2010a, p. 12).

NASN and ANA believe that, in the practice of nursing, competence is definable, is measurable, and can be evaluated. Nonetheless, "no single evaluation method or tool can guarantee competence. Competence is situational, dynamic; it is both an outcome and an ongoing process. Context determines what competencies are necessary" (ANA, 2010a, p. 12).

School nurses are influenced by the nature of the practice situation, which includes consideration of the setting; resources; and the individual, family, group, community, or population. Situations can either enhance or detract from the school nurse's ability to ensure quality care. Competent school nurses promote or facilitate optimal care by altering or adapting to the environmental situation. Competent school nurses strive to influence factors that will facilitate and enhance competent practice. Similarly, competent school nurses deal with barriers that constrain competent practice. The expected level of performance varies depending on the school nursing context and the selected competence framework or model (adapted from ANA, 2010a, p. 13).

According to the "Professional Competency" entry in the NASN *Code of Ethics with Interpretive Statements for the School Nurse* (NASN, 2010b, p. 2), "The school nurse maintains the highest level of competency by enhancing professional knowledge and skills, and by collaborating with peers, other health professionals, and community agencies while adhering to the standards of school nursing practice." An interpretive statement that follows notes, "The profession of nursing is obligated to provide competent nursing care. The school nurse must be aware of the need for continued professional learning and must assume personal responsibility for currency of knowledge and skills."

Definitions and Concepts of Competence

The following apply to competence:

- An individual who demonstrates "competence" is performing successfully at an expected level (ANA, 2010a, p. 12).

- A *competency* is an expected level of performance that integrates knowledge, skills, abilities, and judgment (ANA, 2010a, p. 12).

- The *integration* of *knowledge, skills, abilities,* and *judgment* occurs in *formal, informal,* and *reflective learning* experiences (ANA, 2010a, p. 12).

- *Knowledge* encompasses thinking, understanding of science and humanities, professional standards of practice, and insights gained from practical experiences, personal capabilities, and leadership performance (ANA, 2010a, p. 12).

- *Skills* include psychomotor, communication, interpersonal, and diagnostic skills (ANA, 2010a, p. 12).

- *Ability* is the capacity to act effectively. It requires listening, integrity, knowledge of one's strengths and weaknesses, positive self-regard, emotional intelligence, and openness to feedback (ANA, 2010a, p. 12).

- *Judgment* includes critical thinking, problem-solving, ethical reasoning, and decision-making (ANA, 2010a, p. 13).

- *Formal learning* is a means of integrating knowledge, skills, abilities, and judgment, which most often occurs in structured, academic, and professional development environments, while *informal learning* can be described as experiential insights gained in work, community, home, and other settings (ANA, 2010a, p. 13).

- *Reflective learning* represents recurrent, thoughtful, personal self-assessment, analysis, and the synthesis of strengths and opportunities for improvement. Such insights should lead to the creation of a specific plan for professional development and may become part of one's professional portfolio (ANA, 2010a, p. 13).

Evaluating Competence

Competence in nursing practice must first be evaluated by each school nurse using a self-evaluation process. Then nurse colleagues and nurses in the role of supervisor, coach, mentor, or preceptor can assess the competence of the school nurse. In addition, other aspects of performance not exclusive to the practice of nursing (e.g., interpersonal and communication skills, team collaboration and networking, and classroom teaching) may be evaluated by professional colleagues, administrators, and others. Evaluation should then guide future professional development (adapted from ANA, 2010a, p. 13).

Competence can be evaluated by using tools that capture objective and subjective data about an individual's knowledge and actual performance and that are appropriate for the specific school nursing situation and the desired outcome of the competence evaluation. Such tools and methods include but are not limited to direct observation; records; portfolios; demonstrations; skills lab; performance evaluation; peer review; certification; credentialing; privileging; simulation exercises; computer-simulated and virtual reality testing; targeted continuing education with outcomes measurement; employer skills validation; and practice evaluations (ANA, 2010a, p. 13).

Continuum of School Nursing Practice

School nursing exists on a continuum from generalist to specialist. Because of the broad scope of practice and the complexity of issues addressed by the school nurse, the NASN recommends the minimal educational preparation for a school nurse be a Bachelor of Science in Nursing (BSN) degree from an accredited college or university, as well as state certification in those states requiring or recommending state school nurse licensure/certification. School nurses who have not acquired the BSN degree or state certification credentials are strongly encouraged to meet these qualifications. School nurses must seek professional development and continuing education to increase critical thinking skills and professional judgment, as well as to maintain competence in their role. NASN also recommends that school nurses demonstrate knowledge of school nursing by acquiring certification in the nursing specialty of school nursing. The baccalaureate degree is the minimum level of education required to sit for the national school nurse certification examination. The National Certified School Nurse (NCSN) credential is awarded by the National Board for Certification of School Nurses to those who pass the school nurse certification examination. The credential must be renewed every 5 years through professional development or re-examination, and appropriate documentation must be maintained. In some states, professional development is tied to licensure and recertification. All school nurses have the professional responsibility to maintain their competence in practice.

The continuum of school nurse practice also includes school nurse specialists, such as school nurse consultants, school nurse supervisors and administrators, lead nurses or team leaders, school nurses with advanced clinical preparation, and other specialty roles. School nurses are in lead roles within school districts, charter and private schools, regions, and counties and at the state level. School nurses, as generalists or specialists, focus both on individuals in the community and the population in their practice. Health services are provided within the framework of primary, secondary, and tertiary prevention using epidemiology, biostatistics, and community assessment. Programs and services are offered with the goal of prevention for healthcare consumers.

Statistics of the Profession

As of 2009, there were more than 66,000 practicing school nurses in the United States. Of those, more than 56,000 were in public schools, 5,000 were in private schools, and 5,500 were in other areas of health services (NCES, 2010). In addition, more than 170 school nurses serve healthcare consumers in Department of Defense Education Activity (DoDEA) schools for children of the military (C. Resha, personal communication, September 2010; DoDEA, 2011). Eighty-three percent of school nurses are employed by public school districts, with reported ratios from 1:125 or less to 1:5100 or more (Monsalve, 2010). Membership in the NASN represents 21 percent of all school nurses. In an effort to identify credentialing patterns among members, the NASN conducted a survey with a 19 percent participation rate. Responses indicated that 25 percent of members are nationally certified school nurses. Thirty percent of respondents hold another type of licensure, certification, or credential, such as Advanced Practice Registered Nurse (APRN), certified teacher, or Certified Diabetes Educator. Eighty-three percent of members responding to the NASN survey reported having graduate degrees and 1 percent reported holding doctoral degrees.

Advanced Practice Registered Nurses

Some school nurses may meet the standards identified for APRNs as a result of their education, experience, skill, and authority to practice granted by their state licensing board. APRNs have advanced degrees and national certification in their specialty. In schools, APRNs are nurse practitioners, clinical nurse specialists, or both. They are differentiated by licensure, accreditation of their academic programs, professional specialty certification, and graduate or postgraduate education (APRN Joint Dialogue Group, 2008). APRNs are often part of an enhanced school services team that provides direct diagnostic and treatment care to healthcare consumers. An APRN working in a combined APRN and school nurse role is expected to comply with the standards of practice and professional performance, the associated competencies for all school nurses, and the additional competencies for an APRN. APRNs offer cost-effective solutions to meeting the identified needs of students who do not receive adequate primary care, a major barrier to learning (NASN, 2003).

Graduate-Level Prepared School Nurses

Graduate-level prepared school nurses demonstrate advanced levels of nursing practice that integrate specific, relevant knowledge from school nursing, public health, and other disciplines. These nurses have additional professional experience and graduate-level educational preparation (i.e., master's or doctoral degrees) that support their practice. The advanced education may be in school nursing, administration, education, case management, nursing informatics, public health, research, or other health and nursing areas of study. In graduate programs of study, nurses also advance their knowledge and skills in clinical areas related to the programs, as well as in research.

A graduate-level prepared school nurse is expected to comply with the standards of practice and professional performance for school nursing, the associated competencies for all school nurses, and the additional competencies for a graduate-level prepared school nurse. Resources, such as *Nursing Administration: Scope and Standards of Practice* (ANA, 2009), or *Public Health Nursing: Scope and Standards of Practice* (ANA, 2007b), may provide additional direction.

The practice of the graduate-level prepared school nurse focuses on these:

- *Populations.* Graduate-level prepared school nurses are leaders in population assessment drawing on multiple data sources to synthesize population needs. Many graduate-level prepared nurses have combined job descriptions/responsibilities that often include provision of direct care to students, as well as responsibilities leading population-level care.

- *Systems.* Graduate-level prepared school nurses work in multiple sectors and with multiple disciplines serving the healthcare consumer. They work at a system level and are experts in communications that maximize interactions throughout systems.

- *Complexity.* Graduate-level prepared school nurses are skilled at managing and solving complex, multilevel, and simultaneously occurring problems and issues.

- *Growth of the Specialty.* Graduate-level prepared school nurses assume leadership positions to actively engage in defining, articulating the direction, and advancing the specialty of school nursing. They also evaluate, conduct, and apply evidence-based research to advance the specialty and engage in development of standards and guidelines for school nursing practice.

Roles and Responsibilities of School Nurses

The school nurse role is unique because it encompasses both community health nursing and public health nursing responsibilities. Community health nursing focuses on the individual in the community and subsequently influences the community, while public health nursing focuses on the population and subsequently influences the individual. The combined responsibilities require competencies that are individually focused and focused on population care. "School nursing has a rich history of supporting both education and health missions to promote the health and well-being of children" (Wolfe, in press). More than 100 years ago, public health nurse founder Lillian Wald envisioned a role for the nurse within the community to serve all, regardless of economic or social status or national origin. Unlike the early medical model of public health that initially focused on exclusion of students with infection, the school nursing model has fostered the inclusion of all children in the school setting since its inception. In the 21st century, school nurses continue to support children in meeting the universal goals of education and health for academic success and optimal wellness (Wolfe, in press). "In successful school nursing practice, these goals weave seamlessly together to create a safety net and springboard for children to grow into healthy and successful citizens" (Wolfe, in press).

The healthcare consumer for the school nurse includes not only the student, but also the student's family, the educational employees of the school, the school population at large, and the community. Throughout this document, the term "healthcare consumer" refers to the collective of school nursing clients. There are explicit times when a school nursing standard refers directly to the student only; therefore the term "student" is used.

Key Roles

School nurses deliver services via a variety of delivery modalities such as consultant, direct services delivery, expert resource, and others. Key roles of the school nurse are clinician, advocate, coordinator, case manager, health counselor, health educator, community educator, liaison, researcher, and interprofessional student services team participant. School nurses work with individuals serving children from birth through age 21 (and even older in some states), as well as their families. Their practice is population-focused.

Key Responsibilities

The school nurse is likely to be the only healthcare provider in the broader educational setting. Other healthcare workers, such as occupational therapists or physical therapists, have specific caseloads within the school. The school nurse may be responsible for the entire student population in a given school, district, or identified region. The school nurse collaborates with other health-care professionals to provide successful interventions that result in positive healthcare consumer outcomes. School nurses provide a healthcare safety net for many students by working with healthcare consumers to identify a health-care home, coordinate services, and assure continuity of care. Because school nurses are not always available to provide direct care, they must be fully aware of the applicable laws, regulations, and standards pertaining to the delegation of nursing tasks to others; they are frequently asked to delegate nursing care to teachers, school office staff, classroom assistants, and other UAP. Some states may have laws or regulations in place prohibiting such delegation in the educational setting.

The American Nurses Association (ANA) notes that "registered nurses firmly believe it is their obligation to help improve issues related to healthcare consumer care, health, and wellness" (ANA, 2010a, p. 20). This is clearly evident in the specialty area of school nursing. In today's world, communicable diseases are not the only health-related barriers to education. Some of the issues school nurses must address include child abuse/neglect; domestic and school violence; child and adolescent obesity and inactivity; mental health issues, including suicide and alcohol, tobacco, and other drug use; adolescent pregnancy and parenting; environmental health; physical and emotional disabilities and their consequences; complex physical needs; lack of health insurance coverage; homelessness; poverty; and more.

School nursing is the pivotal profession in continuity of care for student healthcare issues. Much of child health care has shifted to the schools as the healthcare system has been restructured to provide most health care in the community. School nurses use the nursing process as outlined in the accompanying Standards of School Nursing Practice to implement strategies that promote health and safety. They develop team relationships within the school community and with outside providers so that care is coordinated across settings to meet individual health needs and to avoid duplication of efforts and services (ANA, 2007a; NASN, 2002).

Students with Special Needs

A unique role for the nurse in the school is the provision of nursing services to children with disabilities, as well as to those with certain acute or chronic illnesses. The school nurse, alone or with others, develops plans unique to the school setting. Among these are the following:

- The Individualized Healthcare Plan (IHP), the nurse's plan of care for a student with any kind of special need

- The Emergency Care (or Action) Plan (ECP or EAP), the nurse's guide for school staff to facilitate quick and appropriate response in an individual student emergency

- The Individualized Educational Program Plan (IEPP), a multidisciplinary and multifaceted plan for students 5 through 21 years (older in some states) who meet special education program requirements under state and federal law

- The Individual Family Service Plan (IFSP), also a multidisciplinary plan, specific to infants, toddlers, and preschoolers with special needs, and inclusive of their families

- The 504 Accommodation Plan, a multidisciplinary, federally mandated plan to assure physical and other accommodations for children with disabilities

- The transition plan, a multidisciplinary plan designed to facilitate smooth transition among and between schools or school levels for students with special needs

- A crisis management plan, codeveloped by multiple constituencies in preparation for a schoolwide or community disaster or crisis

(Fitzpatrick, 2006; Zimmerman, in press)

Coordinated School Health Program

The school nurse's primary role is to support student learning by addressing concerns that are likely to affect a student's ability to learn. "The coordinated school health initiative has emerged in response to the state of children's health and education. It is an organized set of policies, procedures, and activities designed to protect and promote the health and well-being of the school community" (NASN, 2008). The school nurse provides comprehensive services in all eight components of the Coordinated School Health Program (CSHP), with particular responsibility for managing the school health program. Program management by the school nurse extends from prevention and anticipatory guidance to crisis management and program planning. Specific responsibilities are as diverse as the healthcare consumers and communities served (Thomas, 2006).

The components—health services, health education, environment, nutrition, physical education/activity, counseling/mental health, family/community involvement, and staff wellness—of the CSHP (CDC, 2010a; Marx, Wooley, & Northrop, 1998; Thomas, 2006) are described below:

- *Health Services.* The school nurse serves as the coordinator of the health services program; provides nursing care; advocates for health rights and optimization of health and abilities; and provides referral for services.

- *Health Education.* The school nurse provides appropriate health information and instruction that promotes informed healthcare decisions; promotes health; prevents disease; and enhances school performance.

- *Environment.* The school nurse identifies physical health, emotional health, and safety concerns in the school community; promotes a safe and nurturing school environment; and promotes injury prevention.

- *Nutrition.* The school nurse supports school food service and food-safe schools and promotes the benefits of healthy eating patterns.

- *Physical Education/Activity.* The school nurse promotes healthy activities; physical education; and sports policies/practices that promote safety, good sportsmanship, and a life-long active lifestyle.

- *Counseling/Mental Health.* The school nurse provides health counseling; assesses mental health needs; provides mental health interventions; refers students to appropriate school staff or community agencies; and provides follow-up once treatment is prescribed.

- *Family/Community Involvement.* The school nurse promotes family and community participation in assuring a healthy school and serves as school liaison to families, community groups, and a health advisory committee.

- *Staff Wellness.* The school nurse provides health education and counseling, and promotes healthy activities and environment for school staff.

School Nursing Settings

School nurses are typically employed by local school districts or education systems, although health systems such as public health, hospital, and private health corporations may be the employer. School nursing takes place primarily within local education agencies, serving healthcare consumers, including preschool and school-age children, their families, and members of the school community. However, school nurses also provide services in other locations: juvenile justice centers; alternative treatment centers; preschools; magnet and charter schools; hospital schools; college campuses; learning sites for children of personnel in the armed services; and residential campuses within the larger surrounding community. Care is also provided in students' homes, vocational/occupational settings, and environmental camps; during field trips, school competitions, and sporting events; and, in some cases, also in planning for health care during transportation to and from those venues. In some states, school nurses also provide services to infants and toddlers with disabilities and their families exclusively within their homes.

School-Based Health Centers

Within the educational setting, some states have school-based health centers (SBHCs) in place. The SBHCs were developed in the 1970s to help remove barriers to access to primary care by providing on-site, quality, consistent, and developmentally appropriate services to students. The number of SBHCs has grown significantly in the last four decades. The staff of SBHCs generally provides primary services such as health, dental, mental health, and social services, as well as health education. Advanced practice registered nurses and other graduate-level professionals, such as social workers or nutritionists, often are employed by SBHCs to provide these primary health and social services (NASBHC, 2010). Unlike school nursing services, which are equally available to all students, SBHCs may be limited to certain cohorts of students (for example, students receiving Medicaid) and require an enrollment process to access services.

"While SBHCs do exist in schools with no school nursing services or only limited services, they cannot take their place. In fact, they work best in schools with school nursing services" (NASN, 2001). School nursing services and SBHCs both provide unique and valuable services for children and youth that ultimately facilitate positive outcomes for the school community. The integration of school nursing services and the services of SBHC staff ensures that school-age children and youth will have access to the continuum of health services to support them throughout their educational experience. In some settings, school nurses also deliver services in SBHCs, functioning as both school nurse and APRN.

Science and Art of School Nursing

School nursing is both a science and an art. The *science* of school nursing draws on multiple disciplines, including public health, organization and administrative sciences, and the basic nursing sciences. The *art* of school nursing combines caring, ethics, the personal knowledge and experiences of the nurse, interpersonal relationships, intuition, and the aesthetics of nursing to create holistic nursing practice and enhance the science of nursing (Chinn & Kramer, 2008).

Science of School Nursing

The practice of school nursing is built around sound theory, research, and consensus models of practice drawn from a large body of published work in nursing and school nursing, beginning with Nightingale (1860/1969). The actions of the school nurse focus on strengthening and facilitating students' educational outcomes through the application of theory and the implementation of evidence-based nursing care. Nursing actions are directed to the healthcare consumer (i.e., students and/or those influencing students such as the family, school community, the larger surrounding community, aggregates within the school population, or the entire school population).

The science of school nursing, based on long-established and proven roles, supports the use of standardized language taxonomies, such as those of the North American Nursing Diagnosis Association (NANDA) for nursing diagnosis; Nursing Outcomes Classification (NOC) for nursing outcomes; and Nursing Interventions Classification (NIC) for nursing interventions. Specific nursing interventions, for example, are successful in attaining specific outcomes for school healthcare consumers (Lunney et al., 1997; Lunney, 2006). The italicized interventions that follow have been authenticated by the Center for Nursing Classification and Effectiveness at The University of Iowa and are contained within *Nursing Interventions Classification* (Bulechek, Butcher, & Dochterman, 2007). They are commonly used in school nursing to achieve desired outcomes (Lunney, 2006). School nursing interventions include health promotive efforts, such as *anticipatory guidance, nutritional counseling*, and *exercise promotion*; health education endeavors, such as *smoking cessation assistance, group* (classroom) *teaching*, and *parent education*; preventive health services, such as *infection control, immunization/vaccination management*, and *sports-injury prevention*; health assessment activities, such as *active listening, health screening*, and *environmental management*; the provision of direct nursing care, such as *medication administration, ostomy care, counseling*, and *substance use overdose treatment*; and care coordination, such as *referral, consultation*, and *case management* (Bulechek et al., 2007). Advanced practice registered nurses may also use ICD-9, ICD-10, and CPT as terminologies to support their nursing practice.

The science of school nursing further supports the school nurse as the liaison between the school, family, community healthcare providers, and the school-based or school-linked clinics. The school nurse is the healthcare expert within the school system and the leader in school health policy development, including strategies to evaluate implementation of policies. As the healthcare expert, the school nurse provides leadership in and for the CSHPs, disaster preparedness teams, and the school health advisory councils. NASN (2010c) maintains that the practice of school nursing is unique because of the breadth of practice and because the practice is set in a non-healthcare setting.

The school nurse must demonstrate competency in pediatric and adolescent health assessment, public health, community health, and adult and child mental health nursing. Competencies in health promotion, family assessment, care coordination, communication, program planning, leadership, organization, and time management are essential. To be integrated into the school community, school nurses must be able to interpret the influence of health and education law on student health and learning. The school nurse often is physically isolated from other nursing and healthcare colleagues, and as such, must be comfortable and skilled with independent program management of the health office and the healthcare consumer caseload (Wolfe, 2006).

Art of School Nursing

School nurses also practice the art of nursing. Professional nursing promotes healing and health in a way that builds a relationship between the nurse and the healthcare consumer; incorporates cultural competence; and uses specific processes and practices in providing care (Watson, 1999, 2008; Leininger, 1988; Swanson, 1993).

The essence of nursing is caring. School nurses possess skills and behaviors that support their ability to develop partnerships with healthcare consumers and colleagues, maintain interpersonal relationships, build trust, and demonstrate cultural competence. The school nurse often connects with the healthcare consumer in ways that create environments of acceptance and tolerance. School nurses demonstrate caring throughout their practice by becoming part of the school community and understanding the community needs. School nurses foster independence and self-care in all students and their families and play an essential role in helping students navigate physical and emotional transitions within the educational system as they move from early childhood to adolescence and finally into early adulthood. Last, school nurses practice caring through their image, actions, and moral sensitivity to the individuals and the populations they serve.

Ethical Considerations in School Nursing

The practice of school nursing requires vigilant attention to ethics. The school nurse is an advocate for healthcare consumers. The school nurse provides age-appropriate, culturally, and ethnically sensitive care to healthcare consumers. The school nurse promotes active, informed participation in health decisions; respects the individual's right to be treated with dignity; and understands the ethical and legal issues surrounding an individual's right to privacy and confidentiality. The school nurse treats all members of the school community equally, regardless of race, gender, social or economic status, culture, age, sexual orientation, disability, or religion.

The school nurse maintains the highest level of competency by enhancing professional knowledge and skills; collaborating with peers, other health professionals, and community agencies; and adhering to *Nursing's Social Policy Statement: The Essence of the Profession* (ANA, 2010b), *Code of Ethics for Nurses with Interpretive Statements* (ANA, 2001), *Code of Ethics with Interpretive Statements for the School Nurse* (NASN, 2010b), and this document, *School Nursing: Scope and Standards of Practice, Second Edition*. School nurses participate in the specialty's efforts to advance and use the standards of practice, expand the body of school nursing knowledge through nursing research, and improve conditions of the workplace environment. School nurses are expected to self-regulate as they are responsible to themselves and others for the quality of their practice. The school nurse is autonomous and must engage in personal accountability for quality assurance.

The school nurse practices in an environment that has changed dramatically since the early 20th century. The Individuals with Disabilities Education Act of 1975 [with several subsequent revisions], Section 504 of the Rehabilitation Act of 1973, and the Americans with Disabilities Act of 1990 have contributed to removing barriers that have hindered students' access to education (Gregory, 2006). Education regulations heighten the complexity of decision-making and practice, such as those of the Family Education Rights and Privacy Act (FERPA) of 1974 and subsequent amendments, such as Do Not Resuscitate Orders in the School Setting (AAP, 2010; Kelly, 2006; Marcontel-Shattuck & Gregory, 2006; NASN, 2004). The privacy restrictions to medical information by the Health Information Portability and Accountability Act (HIPAA, 1996) present an ongoing challenge to school nurses who need information about student healthcare needs for the provision of adequate care at school (Kelly, 2006). These laws and regulations influence one aspect of the school nurse's ethical decision-making, necessitating constant updating of knowledge and understanding.

The degree to which the total school community supports school nursing practice affects the delivery of nursing care and, hence, the ethical nature of that care. *Healthy People 2020* advocates a school nurse-to-student ratio of 1:750 in the national health objectives (CDC, 2010b). Inadequate staffing may contribute to the ineffective delivery of care, compromised staff and student wellness, and conflict and stress among school nursing professionals. The appropriateness of this ratio depends on the needs of the school population. In schools in which the population includes a number of children with special needs, 750 students may not be a practical or safe ratio for one school nurse. In addition, school nurses may face ethical challenges when responding to the increased demands in caring for children with complex healthcare needs. Often these children consume much of the school nurse's time and, as such, school nurses may struggle with balancing the needs of children with complex healthcare needs while assuring the school population needs are met. Finally, the recommended ratio may not be applicable or appropriate if geographic distance between schools is such that nurses spend considerable time traveling, resulting in an ethically questionable level of care.

School nurses straddle two statutory and regulatory systems, namely education and health. Because school nurses practice nursing in an education-ally focused system, they face unique policy, funding, and supervisory issues that may also have ethical dimensions. For example, a school request of the school nurse may conflict with nursing practice regulations or a school nurse's responsibilities to the school district may impose restrictions on implementation of nursing practice within the school. As such, school nurses must have not only the skills to communicate within both the healthcare and education arenas, but also the knowledge of the appropriate application of ethical theories and principles.

Summary of the Scope of School Nursing Practice

School nurses continue to adapt their practice to an ever-changing world. New challenges continue to present themselves, as do new tools to assist the school nurse in meeting these challenges. As technology advances, so does the school nurse's practice. More students with more complex daily health needs, as well as those requiring intermittent, on-site nursing treatments, are in schools across America and in Department of Defense Education Activity (DoDEA) schools here and abroad. Technology is available not only as a classroom tool and for expanded school health record keeping, but also to allow students with health impairments greater access to the education they are entitled to receive.

Healthy children are successful learners and children in schools with a Coordinated School Health Program (CSHP) have better educational outcomes (Vinciullo & Bradley, 2009). The school nurse has a multifaceted role within the school setting, one that supports the physical, emotional, mental, and social health of students and their success in the learning process (NASN, 2002). The future of school nursing rests on the ability of the school nurse to successfully meet the challenges in the health and education communities.

School Nursing: Scope and Standards of Practice, Second Edition, delineates the professional responsibilities of all registered school nurses engaged in school nursing practice, regardless of setting. As such it can serve as a basis for a range of uses, such as:

- Position recruitment announcement

- Position description creation

- New employee orientation

- Performance appraisal/evaluation

- Agency policy, protocol, and procedure development

- Competency identification and development

- Education of individuals regarding the role of school nurses

- Quality improvement systems and/or program evaluation efforts

- Development and evaluation of school nursing service delivery systems and organizational structures

- Educational offerings

- Database development, data collection, and research

- Establishing a legal standard

- Healthcare reimbursement and financing methodologies

- Regulatory review and revision

NASN and school nurses support the ANA position regarding the scope and standards of nursing practice, both for all registered nurses and for nursing specialty practitioners: To best serve the public's health and the nursing profession, nursing must continue its efforts to develop its professional standards. Nursing must also examine how such standards can be disseminated and used most effectively to enhance and promote the quality of practice. In addition, such nursing standards must be regularly evaluated as necessary.

The dynamic healthcare practice environment and the growing body of nursing research provide both the impetus and the opportunity for nursing to ensure competent nursing practice in all settings for all healthcare consumers and to promote ongoing professional development that enhances the quality of nursing practice (ANA, 2010a, p. 30).

Standards of School Nursing Practice

The competencies related to each of the standards identify the minimum competencies of all school nurses. Experienced generalist school nurses, however, may perform competencies consistent with advanced education.

The Standards of School Nursing Practice are authoritative statements of the duties that all school nurses are expected to perform competently. The standards published herein may be utilized as evidence of the standard of care, with the understanding that application of the standards is context dependent. The standards are subject to change with the dynamics of the nursing profession and school nursing, as new patterns of professional practice are developed and accepted by the nursing profession, the school nursing community, and the public. In addition, specific conditions and clinical circumstances may also affect the application of the standards at a given time, e.g., during a natural disaster. The standards are subject to formal, periodic review and revision.

The competencies that accompany each standard may be evidence of compliance with the corresponding standard. The list of competencies is not exhaustive. Whether a particular standard or competency applies depends upon the circumstances.

Standards of Practice for School Nursing

Standard 1. Assessment

The school nurse collects comprehensive data pertinent to the healthcare consumer's health and/or the situation.

COMPETENCIES

The school nurse:

- Collects comprehensive data including but not limited to physical, functional, psychosocial, emotional, cognitive, sexual, cultural, age-related, developmental, environmental, spiritual/transpersonal, and economic assessments in a systematic and ongoing process while honoring the uniqueness of the person.

- Elicits healthcare consumers' values, preferences, expressed needs, and knowledge of the healthcare situation.

- Involves the healthcare consumer, family, and other healthcare providers as appropriate, in holistic data collection.

- Identifies barriers (e.g., psychosocial, literacy, financial, cultural) to effective communication and makes appropriate adaptations.

- Recognizes impact of personal attitudes, values, and beliefs.

- Conducts family assessment to include family dynamics, structure, and function.

- Prioritizes data collection activities based on the healthcare consumer's immediate condition or on anticipated needs of the healthcare consumer or situation.

- Uses appropriate evidence-based assessment techniques and instruments and tools.

- Synthesizes available data, information, and knowledge relevant to the situation to identify patterns and variances.

- Applies state and federal legal requirements, ethical standards, and institutional privacy guidelines to the collection, maintenance, use, and dissemination of data and information.

- Recognizes the healthcare consumer as the authority on his/her own health by honoring consumer care preferences.

- Documents relevant data in a retrievable format.

- Uses diagnostic test findings to guide interventions relevant to the healthcare consumer's current status.

- Assesses the effect of interactions among individuals, family, community, and social systems on health and illness.

ADDITIONAL COMPETENCIES FOR THE GRADUATE-LEVEL PREPARED SCHOOL NURSE AND THE ADVANCED PRACTICE REGISTERED NURSE

The graduate-level prepared school nurse or the advanced practice registered nurse:

- Initiates and interprets diagnostic tests and procedures relevant to the healthcare consumer's current status.

- Collects and synthesizes population-focused data from multiple sources throughout the assessment process.

- Partners with populations in need, as well as with relevant health professionals, school colleagues, and other stakeholders to attach meaning to population-focused data.

- Designs a comprehensive data system that focuses on population assets, needs, and concerns in collaboration with public health partners, the population, the interdisciplinary team, and other stakeholders.

- Collaborates with interdisciplinary team to assure maintenance of the data system.

- Evaluates the effectiveness and efficiency of the data system based on current needs with all healthcare partners and consumers.

Standard 2. Diagnosis

The school nurse analyzes the assessment data to determine the diagnoses or issues.

COMPETENCIES
The school nurse:

- Derives the diagnoses or issues through analysis of a broad range of assessment data, including data from the student, family, school staff, and healthcare providers.

- Validates the diagnoses or issues with the healthcare consumer, family, and other healthcare providers when possible and appropriate.

- Identifies actual or potential risks to the healthcare consumer's health and safety or barriers to health, which may include but are not limited to interpersonal, systemic, or environmental circumstances.

- Uses standardized classification systems and clinical decision support tools, when available, in naming diagnoses.

- Documents diagnoses or issues in a retrievable format that facilitates the determination of the expected outcomes and plan.

- Engages in the diagnostic process, including differential diagnosis and the integration and interpretation of various forms of data.

- Bases the analysis on current research and knowledge of clinical diagnoses and normal/abnormal parameters relevant to potential problem areas.

- Selects diagnoses relevant to the school population.

- Explains and interprets the diagnoses or issues to the student and family.

ADDITIONAL COMPETENCIES FOR THE GRADUATE-LEVEL PREPARED SCHOOL NURSE
The graduate-level prepared school nurse:

- Formulates population-based diagnoses as indicated.

- Suggests new or modified diagnoses.

- Considers the interaction of multiple systems in formulating diagnoses.

- Uses complex multisource data in formulating diagnoses.

- Assists nursing staff in maintaining competency in the diagnostic process.

ADDITIONAL COMPETENCIES FOR THE ADVANCED PRACTICE REGISTERED NURSE

The advanced practice registered nurse:

- Systematically compares clinical findings with normal and abnormal variations and developmental events in formulating a differential medical diagnosis.

- Uses complex data and information obtained during interview, examination, and diagnostic processes in identifying medical diagnosis.

Standard 3. Outcomes Identification

The school nurse identifies expected outcomes for a plan individualized to the healthcare consumer or the situation.

COMPETENCIES

The school nurse:

- Involves the student, family, healthcare providers, and others in formulating expected outcomes when possible and appropriate.

- Derives culturally appropriate expected outcomes from the diagnoses.

- Considers associated risks, benefits, costs, current scientific evidence, expected trajectory of the condition, and clinical expertise when formulating expected outcomes.

- Defines expected outcomes in terms of the healthcare consumer, healthcare consumer culture, values and ethical considerations, environment, or situation.

- Includes a time estimate for the attainment of expected outcomes.

- Develops expected outcomes that facilitate continuity of care.

- Modifies expected outcomes based on changes in the status of the healthcare consumer or evaluation of the situation.

- Documents expected outcomes as measurable goals.

- Acts as a resource for the school community in the development of individual health and educational outcomes.

- Uses standardized language or recognizable terminology to document the outcome in a retrievable form.

- Identifies expected outcomes that incorporate scientific evidence and are achievable through implementation of evidence-based practices.

- Identifies expected outcomes that address cost-effectiveness and clinical effectiveness, healthcare consumer satisfaction, and continuity and consistency among providers.

- Differentiates outcomes that require care process interventions from those that require system-level interventions.

ADDITIONAL COMPETENCIES FOR THE GRADUATE-LEVEL PREPARED SCHOOL NURSE AND THE ADVANCED PRACTICE REGISTERED NURSE

The graduate-level prepared school nurse or the advanced practice registered nurse:

- Acts as a resource for the school community in the development of population-based health and educational outcomes.

- Identifies and uses trends in student outcomes to guide district planning for future school programs.

Standard 4. Planning

The school nurse develops a plan that prescribes strategies and alternatives to attain expected outcomes.

COMPETENCIES

The school nurse:

- Develops an individualized plan in partnership with the student and others that considers the student's characteristics or situation, including but not limited to values, beliefs, spiritual and health practices, preferences, choices, developmental level, coping style, culture and environment, and available technology.

- Establishes the plan priorities with the family and others as appropriate.

- Includes in the plan strategies that address each of the identified diagnoses, including emergency care provisions. These strategies may include but are not limited to strategies for promotion and restoration of health; prevention of illness, injury, and disease; the alleviation of suffering; and provision of supportive care for those who are dying.

- Includes strategies for health and wholeness, including complementary and alternative therapies, across the life span.

- Provides for continuity within the plan.

- Incorporates an implementation pathway or timeline within the plan.

- Considers the economic impact of the plan on the healthcare consumer, family, caregivers, or other affected parties, as appropriate to the school setting.

- Integrates current scientific evidence, trends, and research.

- Uses the plan to provide direction to other members of the healthcare team.

- Explores practice settings and safe space and time for the nurse, student, and family to explore suggested, potential, and alternative options.

- Defines the plan to reflect current statutes, rules and regulations, and standards.

- Modifies the plan based on the ongoing assessment of the student's response and other outcome indicators.

- Documents the plan in a manner that uses standardized language or recognized terminology.

- Identifies assessment strategies, diagnostic strategies, and therapeutic interventions that reflect current evidence, including data, research, literature, and expert clinical knowledge.

- Selects or designs strategies to meet the multifaceted needs of students with complex healthcare needs.

- Identifies an evaluation strategy.

- Includes the synthesis of student and family values and beliefs regarding nursing and medical therapies in the plan.

ADDITIONAL COMPETENCIES FOR THE GRADUATE-LEVEL PREPARED SCHOOL NURSE AND THE ADVANCED PRACTICE REGISTERED NURSE

The graduate-level prepared school nurse or advanced practice registered nurse:

- Leads the design and development of interprofessional processes to address the identified diagnosis or issue.

- Actively participates in the development and continuous improvement of systems that support the planning process.

Standard 5. Implementation

The school nurse implements the identified plan.

COMPETENCIES

The school nurse:

- Partners with the student, family, significant others, and caregivers as appropriate to implement the plan in a safe, realistic, and timely manner.

- Demonstrates caring behaviors toward healthcare consumers, significant others, and groups of people receiving care.

- Uses technology to measure, record, and retrieve healthcare consumer data; to implement the nursing process; and to enhance nursing practice.

- Uses evidence-based interventions and treatments specific to the diagnosis or problem.

- Provides holistic care that addresses the needs of diverse populations across the life span.

- Advocates for health care that is sensitive to the needs of healthcare consumers, with particular emphasis on the needs of diverse populations.

- Applies appropriate knowledge of major health problems and cultural diversity in the implementation of the plan of care.

- Applies available healthcare technologies to maximize access and optimal outcomes for healthcare consumers.

- Uses community resources and systems to implement the plan.

- Collaborates with healthcare providers from diverse backgrounds to implement and integrate the plan.

- Accommodates different styles of communication used by healthcare consumers, families, and healthcare providers.

- Integrates traditional and complementary healthcare practices as appropriate.

- Promotes the healthcare consumer's capacity for the optimal level of participation and problem-solving.

- Documents implementation and any modifications, including changes or omissions, of the identified plan in the appropriate health and educational records.

- Provides medically prescribed interventions, including medication administration and medical/nursing treatments, and standard care of ill and injured healthcare consumers in the school community.

- Responds to health issues by providing counseling and crisis intervention when required in such areas as teen pregnancy, substance abuse, death of family members, suicide, and child neglect or abuse.

- Participates, with healthcare consumer direction, in assessing and assuring responsible use of interventions to minimize unwarranted or unwanted treatment and healthcare consumer suffering.

- Coordinates delivery and provides for the continuity of supports and services as identified in the healthcare plan.

- Facilitates utilization of systems, organizations, and community resources to implement the plan.

- Supports collaboration with nursing and other colleagues to implement the plan.

- Incorporates new knowledge and strategies to initiate change in nursing care practices if desired outcomes are not achieved.

- Assumes responsibility for the safe and efficient implementation of the plan.

- Uses communication skills to promote healthy relationships between nurses and healthcare consumers, to provide a context for open discussion of healthcare consumer experiences, and to improve healthcare consumer outcomes.

- Facilitates use of systems, organizations, and community resources to implement the plan.

ADDITIONAL COMPETENCIES FOR THE GRADUATE-LEVEL PREPARED SCHOOL NURSE AND THE ADVANCED PRACTICE REGISTERED NURSE

The graduate-level prepared school nurse or the advanced practice registered nurse:

- Actively participates in the development and continuous improvement of systems that support the implementation of the plan.

- Uses principles and concepts of project or systems management.

- Fosters organizational systems that support implementation of the plan.

- Participates in the development and implementation of written policies and procedures for the clinical services and programs addressing health issues within the school setting.

- Mentors other school nurses on appropriate implementation of plans.

Standard 5A. Coordination of Care

The school nurse coordinates care delivery.

COMPETENCIES

The school nurse:

- Organizes the components of the plan.

- Manages a healthcare consumer's care to maximize independence and quality of life.

- Assists the healthcare consumer in identifying options for alternative care.

- Communicates with the healthcare consumer, family, and system during transitions in care.

- Advocates for the delivery of dignified, culturally competent, developmentally appropriate, and humane care by the interprofessional team.

- Documents coordination of the care.

- Educates colleagues regarding implementation of the plan.

- Incorporates the individualized healthcare plan into the student's educational day and after-school activities.

- Coordinates creation and implementation of the individualized healthcare plan.

ADDITIONAL COMPETENCIES FOR THE GRADUATE-LEVEL PREPARED SCHOOL NURSE AND THE ADVANCED PRACTICE REGISTERED NURSE

The graduate-level prepared school nurse or the advanced practice registered nurse:

- Provides leadership in the coordination of interprofessional health care for integrated delivery of healthcare consumer care services.

- Synthesizes data and information to prescribe necessary education and healthcare system and community support measures, including modifications of surroundings.

- Coordinates education and healthcare system and community resources that enhance delivery of care across continuums.

Standard 5B. Health Teaching and Health Promotion

The school nurse employs strategies to promote health and a safe environment, especially regarding health education.

COMPETENCIES

The school nurse:

- Provides health teaching that addresses such topics as healthy lifestyles, risk-reducing behaviors, developmental needs, activities of daily living, and preventive self-care (as appropriate to developmental needs of the healthcare consumer).

- Uses health promotion and health teaching methods appropriate to the situation and the healthcare consumer's values, beliefs, health practices, developmental level, learning needs, readiness and ability to learn, language preference, spirituality, culture, and socioeconomic status.

- Seeks opportunities for feedback and evaluation of the effectiveness of the strategies used.

- Uses information technologies to communicate health promotion and disease prevention information to the healthcare consumer in a variety of settings.

- Provides healthcare consumers with information about intended effects and potential adverse effects of proposed interventions within the school setting.

- Participates in needs assessment for health education and health instruction for individuals and groups of healthcare consumers.

- Provides general health education to the student body at large through classroom instruction or expert consultation.

- Provides individual and group health teaching and health counseling for and with healthcare consumers.

- Promotes health, wellness, self-care, and safety through education of the school community regarding health issues.

- Designs health information materials and activities for healthcare consumer education appropriate to the consumer's developmental level, learning needs, readiness to learn, and cultural values and beliefs.

- Promotes health principles through the Coordinated School Health Program for all in the school community.

- Evaluates health information resources, such as those available on the Internet, within the area of practice for accuracy, readability, and comprehensibility to help healthcare consumers access quality health information.

- Engages consumer alliances and advocacy groups, as appropriate, in health teaching and health promotion activities.

- Provides anticipatory guidance to individuals, families, groups, and communities to promote health and prevent or reduce the risk of health problems.

- Serves as a primary resource to school staff (and others, as appropriate) regarding health education.

ADDITIONAL COMPETENCIES FOR THE GRADUATE-LEVEL PREPARED SCHOOL NURSE AND THE ADVANCED PRACTICE REGISTERED NURSE

The graduate-level prepared school nurse or the advanced practice registered nurse:

- Synthesizes empirical evidence on risk behaviors, learning theories, behavioral change theories, motivational theories, epidemiology, and other related theories and frameworks when designing health education information materials, activities, and programs.

- Conducts personalized health teaching and counseling considering comparative-effectiveness research recommendations.

- Participates in the evaluation of health curricula and other health instructional materials and activities.

Standard 5C. Consultation

The school nurse provides consultation to influence the identified plan, enhance the abilities of others, and effect change.

COMPETENCIES

The school nurse:

- Seeks consultation with other health professionals.

- Documents consultation with other healthcare providers and other professionals to assure implementation of the plan.

- Synthesizes data according to evidence-based practice and theoretical frameworks when providing consultation.

- Independently communicates recommendations to and facilitates understanding by community-based providers and agencies.

- Facilitates the effectiveness of consultation by involving the healthcare consumers and stakeholders in decision-making and negotiating role responsibilities.

- Communicates consultation recommendations that influence the identified plan, facilitate understanding by stakeholders, enhance the work of others, and effect change.

- Acquires knowledge through participation in formal or informal consultation to address issues in nursing practice.

ADDITIONAL COMPETENCIES FOR THE GRADUATE-LEVEL PREPARED SCHOOL NURSE AND THE ADVANCED PRACTICE REGISTERED NURSE

The graduate-level prepared school nurse or the advanced practice registered nurse:

- Synthesizes data according to evidence-based practice and theoretical frameworks when providing consultation.

- Develops models for effective communication.

- Serves as a mentor and resource to others on effective consultation practices.

- Synthesizes clinical data, theoretical frameworks, and evidence when providing consultation.

Standard 5D. Prescriptive Authority and Treatment

The advanced practice registered nurse uses prescriptive authority, procedures, referrals, treatments, and therapies in accordance with state and federal laws and regulations.

COMPETENCIES FOR THE ADVANCED PRACTICE REGISTERED NURSE

The advanced practice registered nurse:

- Prescribes evidence-based treatments, therapies, and procedures considering the healthcare consumer's comprehensive healthcare needs.

- Prescribes pharmacological agents based on a current knowledge of pharmacology and physiology.

- Prescribes specific pharmacological agents and/or treatments based on clinical indicators, the healthcare consumer's status and needs, and the results of diagnostic and laboratory tests.

- Evaluates therapeutic and potential adverse effects of pharmacological and nonpharmacological treatments.

- Provides healthcare consumers with information about intended effects and potential adverse effects of proposed prescriptive therapies.

- Provides information about costs, alternative treatments, and procedures, as appropriate.

- Evaluates and incorporates complementary and alternative therapy into education and practice.

- Documents all prescriptive interventions, procedures, referrals, treatments, and therapies according to regulatory rules.

Standard 6. Evaluation

The school nurse evaluates progress toward attainment of outcomes.

COMPETENCIES

The school nurse:

- Conducts a systematic, ongoing, and criterion-based evaluation of the outcomes in relation to the structures and processes prescribed by the plan and the indicated timeline.

- Collaborates with the healthcare consumer and others involved in the care or situation in the evaluation process.

- Evaluates, in partnership with the healthcare consumer, the effectiveness of the planned strategies in relation to the healthcare consumer's responses and the attainment of the expected outcomes.

- Uses ongoing assessment data to revise the diagnoses, outcomes, plan, and implementation, as needed.

- Disseminates the results to the healthcare consumer, family, and others involved, in accordance with federal and state regulations.

- Participates in assessing and assuring the responsible and appropriate use of interventions to minimize unwarranted or unwanted treatment and healthcare consumer suffering.

- Documents the results of the evaluation.

- Adapts the plan for the trajectory of treatment based on evaluation of the response.

- Evaluates the accuracy of the diagnosis and effectiveness of the interventions, including complementary and alternative therapies, and other variables in relation to the healthcare consumer's attainment of expected outcomes.

ADDITIONAL COMPETENCIES FOR THE GRADUATE-LEVEL PREPARED SCHOOL NURSE AND THE ADVANCED PRACTICE REGISTERED NURSE

The graduate-level prepared school nurse or the advanced practice registered nurse:

- Synthesizes the results of the evaluation to determine the effect of the plan on healthcare consumers, families, groups, school communities, and institutions.

- Aggregates the data from student healthcare consumer outcomes to effect change to policies and procedures and promote school health programs that support student learning and healthy development.

- Uses the results of the evaluation to make or recommend process or structural changes including policy, procedure, or protocol revision, as appropriate.

Standards of Professional Performance for School Nursing

Standard 7. Ethics

The school nurse practices ethically.

COMPETENCIES

The school nurse:

- Uses *Code of Ethics for Nurses with Interpretive Statements* (ANA, 2001); *Guide to the Code of Ethics for Nurses: Interpretation and Application* (Fowler, 2008); *Code of Ethics with Interpretive Statements for the School Nurse* (NASN 2010b); and other appropriate resources to guide practice.

- Protects the healthcare consumer's autonomy, dignity, rights, values, and beliefs when delivering care.

- Recognizes the centrality of healthcare consumers as core members of any healthcare team.

- Upholds healthcare consumer confidentiality within legal, regulatory, and ethical parameters of health and education.

- Assists healthcare consumers in self-determination and informed decision-making, as developmentally appropriate.

- Maintains a therapeutic and professional healthcare consumer–nurse relationship with appropriate professional role boundaries.

- Contributes to resolving ethical issues involving healthcare consumers, colleagues, community groups, systems, and other stakeholders.

- Takes appropriate action regarding instances of illegal, unethical, or inappropriate behavior that can endanger or jeopardize the best interests of the healthcare consumer or situation.

- Speaks up when appropriate to question healthcare practice when necessary for safety and quality improvement.

- Advocates for equitable healthcare consumer care.

- Participates in interprofessional teams that address ethical risks, benefits, and outcomes.

- Provides information on the risks, benefits, and outcomes of healthcare regimens to allow informed decision-making by the healthcare consumer, including informed consent and informed refusal.

- Integrates caring, kindness, and respect into nursing practice.

ADDITIONAL COMPETENCIES FOR THE GRADUATE-LEVEL PREPARED SCHOOL NURSE AND THE ADVANCED PRACTICE REGISTERED NURSE

The graduate-level prepared school nurse or the advanced practice registered nurse:

- Interprets the risks, benefits, and outcomes of policies, programs, and services for school populations and communities to administrators and others, as well as the potential impact on the delivery of health-related services.

- Partners with multisector team members to address ethical risks, benefits, and outcomes of policies, programs, and services.

- Promotes solutions to social and environmental issues for healthy conditions for the entire school community.

- Acts as a consultant to others to resolve ethical issues of students, colleagues, or systems.

- Contributes to the establishment and operation of an ethics committee for the district.

Standard 8. Education

The school nurse attains knowledge and competence that reflect current nursing practice.

COMPETENCIES

The school nurse:

- Participates in ongoing educational activities related to professional issues.

- Demonstrates a commitment to life-long learning through self-reflection and inquiry to address learning and personal growth needs.

- Acquires knowledge and skills appropriate to the school nursing role; the population of school-age youth, their families, and the school community; and educational settings.

- Seeks formal and independent learning experiences to develop and maintain clinical and professional skills and knowledge.

- Identifies learning needs based on nursing knowledge, the role of the school nurse, and the changing needs of the population within the educational setting.

- Participates in formal and informal consultations to address issues in practice as an application of both an education and a knowledge base.

- Shares educational findings, experiences, and ideas with peers.

- Contributes to a work environment conducive to the education of professionals.

- Maintains professional records that provide evidence of competency and life-long learning.

- Expands clinical knowledge, skills, abilities, and judgment to enhance role performance by incorporating current research.

- Maintains state and national certification and/or credentialing.

ADDITIONAL COMPETENCIES FOR THE GRADUATE-LEVEL PREPARED SCHOOL NURSE AND THE ADVANCED PRACTICE REGISTERED NURSE

The graduate-level prepared school nurse or the advanced practice registered nurse:

- Uses current healthcare research findings and other evidence to expand clinical knowledge, skills, abilities, and judgment for the enhancement of role performance and to increase knowledge of professional issues.

- Uses current healthcare research to plan, design, and implement professional development or higher education programs in school health at the local, state, and national levels.

Standard 9. Evidence-Based Practice and Research

The school nurse integrates evidence and research findings into nursing practice.

COMPETENCIES

The school nurse:

- Uses current evidence-based nursing knowledge, including research findings, to guide practice.

- Incorporates evidence when initiating changes in school nursing practice.

- Participates, as appropriate to education level and position, in the development of evidence-based practice through research activities.

- Shares research findings with colleagues and peers.

- Identifies clinical problems specific to nursing and other research.

- Participates in data collection such as surveys, pilot projects, and formal studies.

- Engages in basic analysis and interpretation of research for application to practice.

- Contributes to the school nursing and school health literature.

- Assures the protection of rights of human subjects in research.

- Complies with school district policy regarding the conduct of research.

- Collaborates with researchers from outside the educational system.

ADDITIONAL COMPETENCIES FOR THE GRADUATE-LEVEL PREPARED SCHOOL NURSE AND THE ADVANCED PRACTICE REGISTERED NURSE

The graduate-level prepared school nurse or the advanced practice registered nurse:

- Contributes to nursing knowledge by conducting or analyzing research and other evidence that identifies, examines, and evaluates knowledge, theories, criteria, and creative approaches to improve healthcare practice.

- Uses research findings in the development of policies, procedures, and standards of care/clinical guidelines.

- Synthesizes research for application to practice.

- Disseminates research findings through activities such as presentations, publications, consultation, and journal clubs.

- Promotes a climate of research and clinical inquiry.

Standard 10. Quality of Practice

The school nurse contributes to quality nursing practice.

COMPETENCIES

The school nurse:

- Demonstrates quality of practice by documenting the application of the nursing process in a responsible, accountable, and ethical manner.

- Uses creativity and innovation to enhance school nursing care.

- Participates in quality improvement activities. Such activities may include:

  - Identifying aspects of practice important for quality monitoring.

  - Using indicators developed to monitor quality and effectiveness of school nursing practice.

  - Collecting data to monitor quality and effectiveness of school nursing practice.

  - Analyzing quality data to identify opportunities for improving school nursing practice.

  - Formulating recommendations to improve school nursing practice or outcomes.

  - Implementing activities to enhance the quality of school nursing practice.

  - Developing, implementing, and evaluating policies, procedures, and/or guidelines to improve the quality of school nursing practice.

  - Participating on and/or leading interprofessional teams to evaluate clinical care or health services.

  - Participating in and/or leading efforts to minimize costs and unnecessary duplication.

  - Identifying problems that occur in day-to-day work routines to correct process inefficiencies.

  - Analyzing factors related to quality, safety, and effectiveness.

- Analyzing organizational systems for barriers to quality healthcare consumer outcomes.

- Implementing processes to remove or decrease barriers within organizational systems.

- Using appropriate tools to monitor the quality and effectiveness of school nursing practice.

ADDITIONAL COMPETENCIES FOR THE GRADUATE-LEVEL PREPARED SCHOOL NURSE AND THE ADVANCED PRACTICE REGISTERED NURSE

The graduate-level prepared school nurse or the advanced practice registered nurse:

- Provides leadership in the design and implementation of quality improvement activities.

- Designs innovations to effect change in school nursing practice to improve health outcomes.

- Evaluates the practice environment and quality of school nursing care rendered in relation to existing evidence.

- Identifies opportunities for the generation and use of research and evidence.

- Obtains and maintains professional certification as a graduate-level prepared school nurse or APRN, if available, in the area of expertise.

- Uses the results of quality improvement activities to initiate changes in school nursing practice and in the healthcare delivery system.

- Synthesizes quality assessment data for program change.

Standard 11. Communication

The school nurse communicates effectively in a variety of formats in all areas of nursing practice.

COMPETENCIES

The school nurse:

- Assesses communication format preferences of healthcare consumers.

- Assesses own communication skills in encounters with healthcare consumers.

- Seeks continuous improvement of own communication and conflict-resolution skills.

- Conveys information to healthcare consumers in formats that promote understanding.

- Questions the rationale supporting care processes and decisions when they do not appear to be in the best interest of the healthcare consumer.

- Discloses observations or concerns related to hazards, errors in care, or the practice environment to the appropriate level of administration.

- Maintains communication with other providers to minimize risks associated with transfers and transition in care delivery.

- Contributes own professional perspective with the multidisciplinary team and others.

- Understands regulations pertaining to privacy and confidentiality to maintain the rights of individual students and families in all communications.

- Uses communication as a strategy to achieve nursing goals.

- Uses effective verbal skills reflective of articulate speech and good listening ability.

- Writes clearly and concisely using correct grammar and spelling.

- Engages in formal health counseling techniques as an effective communication strategy.

ADDITIONAL COMPETENCIES FOR THE GRADUATE-LEVEL PREPARED SCHOOL NURSE AND THE ADVANCED PRACTICE REGISTERED NURSE

The graduate-level prepared school nurse or the advanced practice school nurse:

- Designs districtwide communication systems to meet student and nursing needs.

- Evaluates the effectiveness of districtwide communication systems.

Standard 12. Leadership

The school nurse demonstrates leadership in the professional practice setting and the profession.

COMPETENCIES

The school nurse:

- Oversees the nursing care given by others while retaining accountability for the quality of care given to the healthcare consumer.

- Incorporates the vision and goals of the school organization when planning care, and implementing and measuring progress of an individual student.

- Promotes a commitment to continuous life-long learning and education for self and others.

- Mentors colleagues for the advancement of nursing practice, the profession, and quality healthcare.

- Treats colleagues with respect, trust, and dignity.

- Uses optimal communication and conflict-resolution skills.

- Communicates effectively with the healthcare consumer and colleagues.

- Seeks ways to advance nursing autonomy and accountability of school nurses.

- Participates in efforts to influence school health, public health, and general healthcare policy.

- Participates in school nursing, school health, and other professional organizations.

- Serves in formal and informal leadership roles in professional organizations and committees at local, state, and national levels.

- Participates in committees, councils, or administrative teams in the school or other setting such as school health advisory councils and Section 504 teams.

- Develops a school health advisory committee if one does not exist.

- Shares educational findings, experiences, and ideas with peers to promote a current standard of practice.

- Develops or provides input into the budget for nursing and health services.

- Participates in the design of new nurses' offices, health rooms, or school clinics.

- Mentors colleagues in the acquisition of clinical knowledge, skills, abilities, and judgment.

- Provides peers with formal or informal constructive feedback regarding practice or role performance.

- Provides direction to enhance the effectiveness of the school multidisciplinary team.

- Models expert practice to school multidisciplinary team members and healthcare consumers.

ADDITIONAL COMPETENCIES FOR THE GRADUATE-LEVEL PREPARED SCHOOL NURSE AND THE ADVANCED PRACTICE REGISTERED NURSE

The graduate-level prepared school nurse or the advanced practice registered nurse:

- Promotes advanced practice nursing and role development by interpretation of the role for students, families, and others.

- Shapes the direction of the specialty by actively engaging in such initiatives as development of standards, competencies, role definitions, position statements, and clinical guidelines.

- Analyzes the interaction of systems and their influence on the practice of school nursing.

- Includes a population focus when examining the practice of school nursing.

- Designs and implements performance appraisal systems for school nursing practice.

Standard 13. Collaboration

The school nurse collaborates with the healthcare consumer, family, and others in the conduct of nursing practice.

COMPETENCIES

The school nurse:

- Partners with others to effect change and generate positive outcomes through the sharing of knowledge about the healthcare consumer and/or situation.

- Communicates with healthcare consumers and healthcare providers regarding healthcare consumer care and the school nurse's role in the provision of that care.

- Uses conflict management to facilitate engagement and consensus of strategic partners.

- Participates in building consensus or resolving conflict.

- Applies group process that includes negotiation techniques to maximize collaboration.

- Adheres to standards and applicable codes of conduct that govern behavior among peers and colleagues to create a work environment that promotes cooperation, respect, and trust.

- Cooperates in creating a documented plan focused on outcomes and decisions related to care and delivery of services that reflects communication with healthcare consumers and others.

- Engages in teamwork and team-building processes.

- Functions as a case manager in collaboration with the healthcare consumer and other professionals and agencies.

- Acts as an advocate for the healthcare consumer in multidisciplinary collaboration.

- Functions as a liaison between the family, school, and community.

- Identifies community agencies as possible collaborators or resources.

- Invites the contribution of the student, family, and team members to achieve optimal outcomes.

- Documents the outcomes and decisions of collaborative planning.

ADDITIONAL COMPETENCIES FOR THE GRADUATE-LEVEL PREPARED SCHOOL NURSE AND THE ADVANCED PRACTICE REGISTERED NURSE

The graduate-level prepared school nurse or the advanced practice registered nurse:

- Partners with other disciplines to enhance healthcare consumer outcomes through multidisciplinary activities, such as education, consultation, management, technological development, and policy and program development or research.

- Leads in establishing improved and sustained collaborative relationships for the achievement of safe, quality care for the healthcare consumer.

- Uses knowledge of community health systems and populations to function as an effective collaborator.

- Documents plan-of-care communications, rationales for plan-of-care changes, and collaborative discussions to improve healthcare consumer outcomes.

Standard 14. Professional Practice Evaluation

The school nurse evaluates one's own nursing practice in relation to professional practice standards and guidelines, relevant statutes, rules, and regulations.

COMPETENCIES

The school nurse:

- Provides age-appropriate and developmentally appropriate care in a culturally and ethnically sensitive manner.

- Engages in self-evaluation of practice on a regular basis, identifying areas of strength and areas in which professional development would be beneficial.

- Obtains informal feedback regarding his or her own practice from healthcare consumers, peers, professional colleagues, and others.

- Participates in peer review, as appropriate.

- Takes action to achieve goals identified during the evaluation process.

- Provides evidence for practice decisions and actions as part of the informal and formal evaluation processes.

- Interacts with peers and colleagues to enhance one's own professional nursing practice or role performance.

- Provides peers with formal or informal constructive feedback regarding their practice or role performance.

- Appraises use of developmentally appropriate, culturally and ethnically sensitive care in self-evaluation.

- Engages in a formal process seeking feedback regarding one's own practice from healthcare consumers, peers, professional colleagues, and others.

- Enhances one's own professional nursing practice or role performance by networking and interacting with peers and colleagues.

- Demonstrates achievement of goals identified during the evaluation process.

- Uses recognized and accepted tools in self-evaluation and peer evaluation.

- Takes corrective action to rectify a mistake and reduce future errors.

- Maintains professional responsibility, accountability, and behavior.

Standard 15. Resource Utilization

The school nurse utilizes appropriate resources to plan and provide nursing services that are safe, effective, and financially responsible.

COMPETENCIES
The school nurse:

- Identifies appropriate resources for assessed healthcare consumer care needs and desired outcomes.

- Identifies healthcare consumer care needs, potential for harm, complexity of the task, and desired outcomes when considering resource allocation.

- Delegates elements of care to appropriate healthcare workers, or others, in accordance with any applicable legal or policy parameters or principles.

- Uses available evidence when evaluating resources.

- Advocates for resources, including technology, that enhance school nursing practice and healthcare delivery.

- Adapts resources, including technology, to modify practice in order to promote a positive interface between healthcare consumers and care providers.

- Assists the healthcare consumer in securing appropriate available services, addressing needs across the healthcare continuum such as State Child Health Insurance Programs.

- Assists healthcare consumers in becoming informed consumers about the options, costs, risks, and benefits of health promotion, health education, school health services, and individualized health interventions.

- Evaluates safety, effectiveness, availability, costs, and benefits of resources that would result in the same desired outcomes when choosing among practice options.

- Develops innovative solutions for healthcare consumer problems that address effective resource utilization and maintenance of quality care.

- Documents all aspects of resource utilization, including delegation and staff training.

- Identifies absent or deficient community resources that could enhance the provision of safe and effective healthcare.

- Uses organizational and community resources to formulate multidisciplinary plans of care.

- Develops innovative solutions and applies strategies to obtain appropriate resources for nursing initiatives.

ADDITIONAL COMPETENCIES FOR THE GRADUATE-LEVEL PREPARED SCHOOL NURSE AND THE ADVANCED PRACTICE REGISTERED NURSE

The graduate-level prepared school nurse or the advanced practice registered nurse:

- Designs evaluation strategies to demonstrate safety and effectiveness of interventions and outcomes, cost-effectiveness, cost-benefit, and efficiency factors associated with nursing practice.

- Develops organizational resources to ensure a work environment conducive to completing the identified plan and outcomes.

Standard 16. Environmental Health

The school nurse practices in an environmentally safe and healthy manner.

COMPETENCIES

The school nurse:

- Attains and maintains current knowledge of environmental health concepts, such as implementation of environmental health strategies.

- Promotes a practice environment that reduces environmental health risks of healthcare consumers, including visitors.

- Facilitates the assessment of the practice environment for factors that negatively affect health in the school setting, including safe staffing ratios, food safety, sound, odor, chemicals, mold, noise, and light.

- Advocates for the judicious and appropriate use of products used in the school setting, such as cleaning agents, building materials, and pesticides.

- Assures communication regarding environmental health risks and exposure reduction strategies to student healthcare consumers, families, colleagues, and communities.

- Uses scientific evidence to determine whether a product or treatment is a potential environmental threat.

- Participates in strategies that promote emotionally and physically healthy communities.

- Initiates strategies that promote an emotionally healthy school culture.

- Creates partnerships that promote sustainable environmental health policies, including efforts to promote access to healthy foods and physical activity.

- Critically evaluates environmental health issues that are presented by the popular media.

- Advocates for implementation of environmental health principles in school nursing practice.

ADDITIONAL COMPETENCIES FOR THE GRADUATE-LEVEL PREPARED SCHOOL NURSE AND THE ADVANCED PRACTICE REGISTERED NURSE

The graduate-level prepared school nurse or the advanced practice school nurse:

- Analyzes the impact of social, political, and economic influences on the environment and human health exposures.

- Supports nurses in advocating for and implementing environmental health principles in school nursing practice.

- Designs environmental health programs with interdisciplinary experts to assure a healthy and safe environment.

Standard 17. Program Management

The school nurse manages school health services.

COMPETENCIES

The school nurse:

- Manages school health services as appropriate to the nurse's education, experience, position, and practice environment.

- Conducts health needs assessments of the healthcare consumer to identify current health problems and identify the need for new programs.

- Implements needed health programs using a program planning process.

- Demonstrates knowledge of existing school health programs and current health trends that may affect healthcare consumer care; the sources of funds for each; and local, state, and federal laws governing each.

- Evaluates ongoing health programs for outcomes and quality of care.

- Communicates findings of evaluation of outcomes and care to administrators and the board of education.

- Supervises health assistants, aides, and unlicensed assistive personnel (UAPs), as appropriate and legal in the school setting, to include orientation, training, and documentation of competency.

- Interprets the role of the school nurse and school health service needs to the school and community.

- Participates in the development of an emergency plan that is communicated to the school community.

- Serves on school and district health and wellness committees.

- Acts as a resource for coordinated school health programs.

- Adopts available technology appropriate to the work setting.

- Apprises administration and the superintendent or board of education about the status of the school health program.

- Identifies potential funding sources for nursing and health services.

- Leverages cooperation between schools and communities on public health issues.

ADDITIONAL COMPETENCIES FOR THE GRADUATE-LEVEL PREPARED SCHOOL NURSE AND THE ADVANCED PRACTICE REGISTERED NURSE

The graduate-level prepared school nurse or the advanced practice school nurse:

- Initiates changes throughout the healthcare delivery system, as appropriate, using the results of school health environmental needs assessments, analysis of evaluation data, and quality-of-care activities.

- Develops health policies and procedures in collaboration with the school administration, the board of health, and the board of education.

- Assures implementation of health policies and procedures.

- Leads public health efforts across the school community.

Glossary

Ability. A characteristic of nursing competency that describes the capacity to act effectively. It requires listening, integrity, knowledge of one's strengths and weaknesses, positive self-regard, emotional intelligence, and openness to feedback.

Advanced practice registered nurse (APRN). A nurse who has completed an accredited graduate-level education that prepares her or him for the role of certified nurse practitioner, certified registered nurse anesthetist, certified midwife, or clinical nurse specialist; has passed a national certification examination that measures the APRN role and population-focused competencies; maintains continued competence as evidenced by recertification; and is licensed to practice as an APRN.

Assessment. The first step of the nursing process in which data about the healthcare consumer are systematically and comprehensively collected and analyzed to formulate a nursing diagnosis or diagnoses.

Competence. The state of having the knowledge, judgment, skills, energy, experience, and motivation required to respond safely, effectively, and appropriately to nursing performance expectations and professional responsibilities (Roach, 2002). Competence is definable and measurable and can be evaluated. An individual who demonstrates competence is performing successfully at an expected level.

Competency. An expected level of performance that integrates knowledge, skills, abilities, and judgment, based on established scientific knowledge and expectations for nursing practice. Competency statements are specific, measurable elements that interpret, explain, and facilitate practical use of the standard.

Complexity. An attribute that represents multifactorial influence on a problem or solution; the synthesis of influences and simultaneously occurring problems and issues for effective intervention.

Delegation. The assignment of the performance of a nursing activity to a non-nurse. Accountability remains with the registered nurse; state laws and regulations and school regulations must be followed; and standards of school nursing practice must be upheld.

Diagnosis. The second step of the nursing process in which the analysis of assessed data results in a clinical judgment expressed as a statement of the healthcare consumer's response to actual or potential health needs or conditions. The diagnosis provides the basis for determining a plan to achieve expected outcomes.

Evaluation. The sixth and final step of the nursing process in which the nurse systematically and continuously appraises progress toward attainment of outcomes; measurable elements that interpret, explain, and facilitate practical use of the standard.

Formal learning. A means of integrating knowledge, skills, abilities, and judgment, which most often occurs in structured, academic, and professional development environments.

Graduate-level prepared school nurse. A nursing leader in school nursing and health who possesses specialized knowledge and skills in school nursing, public health, organization and management, health education, health promotion, administration, or other areas of study necessary to advance the health of the healthcare consumer and who has additional professional experience and graduate-level degrees (i.e., master's or doctoral degrees).

Health care. The prevention, treatment, and management of illness; the preservation of mental and physical well-being; and the promotion of health through the services offered by a healthcare provider or health professional.

Healthcare consumer. The individual, family, group, community, or population who is the focus of attention and to whom the school nurse is providing services as sanctioned by state regulatory bodies. The term "healthcare consumer" refers to a collective of school nursing clients.

Healthcare provider. A person licensed to provide direct care to individuals, including diagnosis and treatment of acute and chronic health problems.

Healthy work environment. An employment atmosphere characterized by optimal physical, psychological, economic, and political conditions conducive to optimal productivity, including worker and healthcare consumer safety, employer support and encouragement, absence of undue stress, and reasonable and sustainable staffing conditions and caseloads.

Implementation. The fifth step of the nursing process in which the nurse acts to bring about the plan. In the standards of practice, the process of implementation has several components that include coordination of care; health teaching and health promotion; consultation; and, for the APRN, prescriptive authority and treatment.

Informal learning. A means of integrating knowledge, skills, abilities, and judgment into experiential insights gained in work, community, home, and other settings.

Interprofessional. Reliant on the overlapping knowledge, skills, and abilities of each professional team member. This can drive synergistic effects by which outcomes are enhanced and become more comprehensive than a simple aggregation of the individual efforts of the team members.

Judgment. A characteristic of nursing competency that includes critical thinking, problem-solving, ethical reasoning, and decision-making.

Knowledge. A characteristic of nursing competency that encompasses thinking, understanding of science and humanities, professional standards of practice, and insights gained from practical experiences, personal capabilities, and leadership performance.

Liaison. A person whose function it is to maintain communication between or among individuals and an organization, parts of an organization, or between two or more organizations acting together for a common purpose.

Multidisciplinary team. A team of school or community professionals with a variety of skills, abilities, and disciplinary backgrounds who work together for a common purpose. In the context of the school, this goal is to achieve the best academic and/or health outcomes for students, their families, or other healthcare consumers.

National Association of School Nurses (NASN). A professional organization serving the needs of school nurses nationally and internationally. As such, the NASN supports the health and educational success of children and youth by developing and providing leadership to advance school nursing practice by specialized registered nurses. As the expert voice for school nurses, the organization has as its core values: scholarship; excellence; collegiality; and diversity.

Nursing process. A circular, continuous, and dynamic critical-thinking process comprised of six steps and that is client-centered, interpersonal, collaborative, and universally applicable. The six steps are assessment, diagnosis, outcomes identification, planning, implementation, and evaluation. The nursing process encompasses all significant actions taken by registered nurses and forms the foundation of the school nurse's decision-making.

Outcomes identification. The third step of the nursing process wherein measurable, expected, realistic, and attainable expectations for the healthcare consumer are stipulated.

Planning. The fourth step of the nursing process in which the nurse formulates a comprehensive outline of care to be implemented for attainment of specific measurable outcomes. In school nursing, examples are the Individualized Healthcare Plan (IHP), the Americans with Disabilities Act (504 Plan), the

Individualized Educational Program Plan (IEPP) from the Individuals with Disabilities in Education Act, the Emergency Care Plan (ECP), and others.

Population. Includes aggregates, persons with identified similarities, and communities.

Reflective learning. A means of integrating knowledge, skills, abilities, and judgment brought about through recurrent, thoughtful, personal self-assessment; analysis; and the synthesis of strengths and opportunities for improvement. Such insights should lead to the creation of a specific plan for professional development and may become part of one's professional portfolio.

School. An institution, organization, or group dedicated to the provision of educational services for children and youth from birth through age 21 or older. Schools include public, private, and military entities.

School community. All those who study, work in, or are formally affiliated with a school district or school setting. The school community is expanded, when appropriate, to community agencies, faith-based groups, students' families, and others.

School nurse administrator. A professional registered school nurse who also is recognized or employed in the capacity of supervision of school nurses or others and expected to carry out school health or other administrative responsibilities in the school setting, such as coordination of school health services across the school district, development of school health policies and procedures, establishment of professional development for school nurses, development of school health budgets, and evaluation of school health programs.

School nursing. A specialized practice of professional nursing that advances the well-being, academic success, and life-long achievement and health of students. To that end, school nurses facilitate positive student responses to normal development; promote health and safety, including a healthy environment; intervene with actual and potential health problems; provide case management services; and actively collaborate with others to build student and family capacity for adaptation, self-management, self-advocacy, and learning.

Scope of school nursing practice. A statement describing the complex and unique practice of the school nurse, including its considerable depth and breadth. The scope statement describes the "who," "what," "where," "when," "why," and "how" of school nursing practice. The statement is intended for those who practice school nursing in the United States and its territories, and in Department of Defense Education Activity (DoDEA) locations around the world.

Skills. A characteristic of nursing competency that includes psychomotor, communication, interpersonal, and diagnostic skills.

Standards. Authoritative statements of the duties that all registered nurses, regardless of role, population, or specialty, are expected to perform. Within school nursing, standards are the professional expectations that guide the practice of school nursing.

System. Any group of interacting, interrelated, or interdependent elements forming a complex whole.

Unlicensed assistive personnel (UAP). A person who has been delegated certain appropriate, routine, standardized nursing tasks by a registered nurse, who, after assessment of the individual's capabilities, makes a prudent decision regarding the advisability of delegation. The registered nurse may decide against delegation for safety, regulatory, and legal issues; school staffing or student health status issues; or UAP competence or ability.

References
and Bibliography

All URLs were current when retrieved on May 7, 2011.

American Academy of Pediatrics (AAP), Committee on School Health and Committee on Bioethics. (2010). *Do not resuscitate orders in schools.* Retrieved from http://aappolicy.aappublications.org/cgi/content/full/pediatrics;105/4/878

American Association of Critical-Care Nurses (AACN). (2005). *AACN standards for establishing and sustaining healthy work environments: A journey to excellence.* Mission Viejo, CA: Author.

American Nurses Association (ANA). (1983). *Standards of school nursing practice.* Kansas City, MO: Author.

American Nurses Association (ANA). (2001). *Code of ethics for nurses with interpretive statements.* Silver Spring, MD: Nursesbooks.org.

American Nurses Association (ANA). (2007a). *ANA's principles of environmental health for nursing practice with implementation strategies.* Silver Spring, MD: Nursesbooks.org.

American Nurses Association (ANA). (2007b). *Public health nursing: Scope and standards of practice.* Silver Spring, MD: Nursesbooks.org.

American Nurses Association (ANA). (2009). *Nursing administration: Scope and standards of practice.* Silver Spring, MD: Nursesbooks.org.

American Nurses Association (ANA). (2010a). *Nursing: Scope and standards of practice* (2nd ed.). Silver Spring, MD: Nursesbooks.org.

American Nurses Association (ANA). (2010b). *Nursing's social policy statement: The essence of the profession.* Silver Spring, MD: Nursesbooks.org.

APRN Joint Dialogue Group. (2008). *Consensus model for APRN regulation: Licensure, accreditation, certification, and education.* Retrieved from http://www.nursingworld.org/DocumentVault/APRN-Resource-Section/ ConsensusModelforAPRNRegulation.aspx

Bulechek, G., Butcher, H., & Dochterman, J. M. (2007). *Nursing interventions classification (NIC)* (5th ed.). St. Louis, MO: Mosby.

Centers for Disease Control and Prevention (CDC), National Center for Chronic Disease Prevention and Health Promotion. (2010a). *Coordinated school health.* Retrieved from http://www.cdc.gov/HealthyYouth/CSHP

Centers for Disease Control and Prevention (CDC), National Center for Health Statistics. (2010b). *Healthy people 2020: Education and community-based programs objectives*, ECB5. Retrieved from http://healthypeople.gov/2020/topicsobjectives2020/ objectiveslist.aspx?topicid=11

Chinn, P., & Kramer, M. K. (2008). *Integrated theory and knowledge development in nursing* (7th ed.). St. Louis, MO: Mosby.

Connecticut State Department of Education (CSDE), School Nursing Task Force [C. Resha, chair]. (2009). *Competency in school nurse practice.* Hartford, CT: Author. Retrieved from http://www.sde.ct.gov/sde/lib/sde/ PDF/deps/student/health/Nursing_Competencies.pdf

Department of Defense Education Activity (DoDEA). (2011). Home page. Retrieved from http://www.dodea.edu/home/

Fitzpatrick, B. (2006). Emergency management, crisis response, and the school nurse's role. In J. Selekman (Ed.), *School nursing: A comprehensive text* (pp. 205–233). Philadelphia: F.A. Davis.

Fowler, M. D. M. (Ed.). (2008). *Guide to the code of ethics for nurses: Interpretation and application.* Silver Spring, MD: Nursesbooks.org.

Gallagher-Lepak, S., & Kubsch, S. (2009). Transpersonal caring: A nursing practice guideline. *Holistic Nursing Practice, 23,* 171–172.

Garcia, A. (2009). Dear Lillian: Convincing my school district to lower the school nurse to student ratio to 1:750. *NASN School Nurse, 24*(5), 198.

Gregory, E. K. (2006). Federal laws protecting children and youth with disabilities. In J. Selekman (Ed.), *School nursing: A comprehensive text* (pp. 301–321). Philadelphia: F.A. Davis.

Hagerty, B. M. K., Lynch-Sauer, J., Patusky, K. L., & Bouwsema, M. (1993). An emerging theory of human relatedness. *Journal of Nursing Scholarship, 25*(4), 291–296.

Health Information Portability and Accountability Act of 1996, 42 U.S.C. §1320d-9. (1996). Retrieved from https://www.cms.gov/HIPAAGenInfo/Downloads/HIPAALaw.pdf

Institute of Medicine (IOM). (2004). *Damp indoor spaces and health.* Washington, DC: The National Academies Press. Retrieved from http://www.nap.edu/catalog.php?record_id=11011

Joint Committee of the National Education Association and the American Medical Association. (1941). *The nurse in the school.* Washington, DC: National Education Association and American Medical Association.

Kelly, L. (2006). Legislation affecting school nurses. In J. Selekman (Ed.), *School nursing: A comprehensive text* (pp. 283–300). Philadelphia: F.A. Davis.

Leininger, M. (1988). Leininger's theory of nursing: Cultural care diversity and universality. *Nursing Science Quarterly, 1*(4), 152–160.

Lunney, M. (2006). NANDA diagnoses, NIC interventions, and NOC outcomes used in an electronic health record with elementary school children. *Journal of School Nursing, 22*(2), 94–101.

Lunney, M., Cavendish, R., Luise, B. K., & Richardson, K. (1997). Relevance of NANDA and health promotion diagnoses to school nursing. *Journal of School Nursing, 13*(5), 16–22.

Marcontel-Shattuck, M., & Gregory, E. K. (2006). Dealing with controversy in the practice of school nursing. In J. Selekman (Ed.), *School nursing: A comprehensive text* (pp. 1133–1142). Philadelphia: F.A. Davis.

Marx, E., Wooley, S., & Northrop, D. (1998). *Health is academic*. New York: Teachers College Press.

Monsalve, L. (2010). 2009 membership survey: Developing and providing leadership to advance the school nursing practice. *NASN School Nurse, 25*(4), 176–180.

National Assembly of School-Based Health Centers (NASBHC). (2010). *About school-based health care.* Retrieved from http://www.nasbhc.org/site/c.jsJPKWPFJrH/b.2561553/k.843D/about_sbhcs.htm

National Association of School Nurses (NASN). (2001). *The role of the school nurse in school-based health centers* (position statement). Silver Spring, MD: Author. Retrieved from http://www.nasn.org/Default.aspx?tabid=245

National Association of School Nurses (NASN). (2002). *School nursing services role in healthcare: Role of the school nurse* (issue brief). Silver Spring, MD: Author. Retrieved from http://www.nasn.org/Default.aspx?tabid=279

National Association of School Nurses (NASN). (2003). *The role of the advanced practice registered nurse in the school setting* (position statement). Silver Spring, MD: Author. Retrieved from http://www.nasn.org/Default.aspx?tabid=197

National Association of School Nurses (NASN). (2004). *Do not resuscitate* (position statement). Silver Spring, MD: Author. Retrieved from http://www.nasn.org/Default.aspx?tabid=217

National Association of School Nurses (NASN). (2005). *Environmental impact concerns in the school setting* (position statement). Silver Spring, MD: Author. Retrieved from http://www.nasn.org/Default.aspx?tabid=270

National Association of School Nurses (NASN). (2008). *Coordinated school health programs* (position statement). Silver Spring, MD: Author. Retrieved from http://www.nasn.org/Default.aspx?tabid=213

National Association of School Nurses (NASN). (2010a). *Caseload assignments* (position statement). Silver Spring, MD: Author. Retrieved from http://www.nasn.org/Default.aspx?tabid=209

National Association of School Nurses (NASN). (2010b). *Code of ethics with interpretive statements for the school nurse* [online and brochure]. Silver Spring, MD: Author. Retrieved from http://www.nasn.org/Default.aspx?tabid=512

National Association of School Nurses (NASN). (2010c). Definition of school nursing. *About us* [data file]. Silver Spring, MD: Author. Retrieved from http://www.nasn.org/Default.aspx?tabid=57

National Center for Education Statistics (NCES), U.S. Department of Education, Institute of Educational Sciences. (2010). Public school staff: Appendix A, supplemental table to indicator 30, Table A-30-1 [2007–2008 data]. *The condition of education.* Washington, DC: Author. Retrieved from http://nces.ed.gov/pubsearch/pubsinfo.asp?pubid=2010028

National Education Association (NEA), Department of School Nurses. (1970). *Standards for school nurse services.* Washington, DC: Author.

New Mexico Public Education Department (NMPED). (2008). *Attachments for school nurse evaluation tools* (following pp. I–11). Retrieved from http://www.nmschoolhealthmanual.org

Nightingale, F. (1860/1969). *Notes on nursing: What it is and what it is not.* New York: Dover Publications.

Proctor, S. (In press). Standards of practice: What they are and how to use them. In J. Selekman (Ed.), *School nursing: A comprehensive text* (2nd ed.). Philadelphia: F.A. Davis.

Roach, M. S. (2002). *Caring, the human mode of being: A blueprint for the health professions* (2nd ed.). Ottawa, Ontario, Canada: CHA Press (Presses de l'ACS).

Struthers, L. R. (1917). *The school nurse.* New York: G.P. Putnam's Sons, Knickerbocker Press.

Swanson, K. (1993). Empirical development of a middle-age theory of caring. *Nursing Research, 40*(3), 161–166.

Thomas, E. L. (2006). Coordinated school health programs. In J. Selekman (Ed.), *School nursing: A comprehensive text* (pp. 45–55). Philadelphia: F.A. Davis.

United States Environmental Protection Agency (U.S. EPA). (2010a). *Healthy school environments assessment tool (HealthySEAT).* Retrieved from http://www.epa.gov/schools/healthyseat/index.html

United States Environmental Protection Agency (U.S. EPA). (2010b). *School siting guidelines*. Retrieved from http://www.epa.gov/schools/siting/

Vinciullo, F., & Bradley, B. (2009). A correlational study of the relationship between a coordinated school health program and school achievement: A case for school health. *The Journal of School Nursing, 25*(6), 453–465.

Watson, J. (1999). *Postmodern nursing and beyond*. Edinburgh: Churchill Livingston.

Watson, J. (2008). *Nursing: The philosophy and science of caring*. Boulder, CO: University Press of Colorado.

Wolfe, L. (2006). Roles of the school nurse. In J. Selekman (Ed.), *School nursing: A comprehensive text* (pp. 111–127). Philadelphia: F.A. Davis.

Wolfe, L. (In press). The profession of school nursing. In J. Selekman (Ed.), *School nursing: A comprehensive text* (2nd ed.). Philadelphia: F.A. Davis.

Zimmerman, B. (In press). Student health and education plans. In J. Selekman (Ed.), *School nursing: A comprehensive text* (2nd ed.). Philadelphia: F.A. Davis.

Appendix A.

The Development of School Nursing Standards: Foundational Documents, 1900s to Present

The history of school nursing standards of practice is nearly as long as the history of the specialty itself. Publications by several individuals and organizations trace a developmental trajectory of nearly 100 years during which consensus documents of the school nurse role and function proved fundamental to the development of future standards of practice and professional performance.

The National Association of School Nurses (NASN) has been leading the development of the standards for this specialty in recent decades. During the mid-20th century, however, other groups and individuals played key roles in generating documents that articulated a comprehensive school nursing role. These works contributed significantly to the thinking that culminated in the development of the first set of universally endorsed standards of practice for school nursing. Some of these seminal works are listed in the following table. Committee chairs, authors, and editors are noted when known.

A Timeline of the Development of School Nursing Standards

1917   The first "textbook" of school nursing, *The School Nurse*, is published. Lina Rogers Struthers, the first U.S. school nurse, is the author. Struthers preceded her book with several articles on school nursing published in *The American Journal of Nursing*, one as early as 1903.

1920s–
1950s   **National Organization for Public Health Nursing** (NOPHN) publishes numerous statements on the role, function, and preparation of the public health nurse in the school.

1930s–
1970s   Textbooks about school nursing are published.
             1931–*School Nursing* (Mary Ella Chayer, author).
             1953–*School Nursing in the Community Program* (Marie Swanson, author).
             1963–*The Nurse in the School Health Program* (Gertrude Cromwell, author).
             1973–*School Nursing in Transition* (Doris Bryan, author).

1956   **American Public Health Association** (APHA), Committee on School Nursing, publishes *Cooperative Formulations of School Nurse Functions.*

1956, 1959 **American School Health Association** (ASHA), Committee on School Nursing Policies and Practices, publishes two editions of *Recommended Policies and Practices for School Nursing* (Eunice Lamona, Lyda Smiley, and Irma Fricke, co-committee chairs).

1955, 1961, **American Nurses Association**, School Nurses Branch, publishes
1966   three editions of *Functions, Standards, and Qualifications of School Nurses.*

1963   *Evaluation of School Nursing Activities: A Pilot Project Using a Scoring System and Accepted Standards of School Nursing* is published (Delores Basco, Supervising Public Health Nurse, Baltimore City Health Department, author).

1967   **American School Health Association** publishes *The Nurse in the School Health Program: Guidelines for School Nurses.*

1969   **National Council of School Nurse Organizations** publishes *The Unique Functions of the Professional School Nurse.*

1970   **Department of School Nurses** (DSN, later NASN) **of the National Education Association** (NEA) publishes *Standards for School Nurse Services* (Gemma Jean, committee chair).

1970–Present   **Department of School Nurses/National Association of School Nurses** publishes *School Nurse,* later *The Journal of School Nursing,* and the *NASN Newsletter,* later *NASN School Nurse;* the **American School Health Association** publishes *The Journal of School Health.*

1973   **American Nurses Association** publishes the first "generic" standards for all of nursing: *Standards of Nursing Practice* with subsequent revisions in 1991, 1998, 2004, and 2010.

1974   **American School Health Association's** School Nurse Section revises earlier work and publishes *Guidelines for the School Nurse in the School Health Program* (Virginia Thompson, committee chair).

1981   *School Nursing: A Framework for Practice* is published (Susan Wold, editor and contributing author).

1981, 1990   **National Association of School Nurses** publishes *Guidelines for the Model School Nurse Services Program* (Helen Weber, committee chair). The book was revised and updated nine years later (Susan Proctor, author).

1983   **American Nurses Association** publishes the first interorga-
nizationally developed and endorsed practice standards for
school nursing: *Standards of School Nursing Practice* (Georgia
Macdonough, committee chair).

1991   **American School Health Association** publishes an implemen-
tation guide for the 1983 standards of practice: *Implementation
Guide for the Standards of School Nursing Practice* (Alicia
Snyder, editor and committee chair).

1993   **National Association of School Nurses** publishes an imple-
mentation guide for 1983 standards of practice: *School Nursing
Practice: Roles and Standards* (Susan Proctor, author, with
Susan Lordi and Donna Zaiger).

1998   **National Association of School Nurses and American Nurses
Association** publish the next edition of the school nursing stan-
dards: *Standards of Professional School Nursing Practice* (Charla
Dunham, committee chair).

2000   **National Association of School Nurses** publishes an implementation guide for the 1998 standards: *Standards of Professional
School Nursing Practice: Applications in the Field* (Susan Lordi,
author, with Beverly Bradley).

2001   **National Association of School Nurses and American Nurses
Association** republish the 1998 standards with no changes
but with the addition of a "scope of practice" statement: *Scope
and Standards of Professional School Nursing Practice* (Charla
Dunham, committee chair).

2005   **National Association of School Nurses and American Nurses
Association** publish the next edition of school nursing standards:
School Nursing: Scope and Standards of Practice (Elizabeth
"Libby" Thomas, committee chair and editor).

2006, 2012   *School Nursing: A Comprehensive Text* is first published in 2006 (Janice Selekman, editor and contributing author). (Its second edition is scheduled for publication in January 2012.)

2011   **National Association of School Nurses and American Nurses Association** publish *School Nursing: Scope and Standards of Practice* (2nd ed.)* (Elizabeth "Libby" Thomas, committee chair).

* The 2011 revision, while the second edition with this title, is also the fifth iteration of a sequence of published standards: 1983; 1998; 2001; 2005; 2011.

Appendix B.

School Nursing: Scope and Standards of Practice (2005)

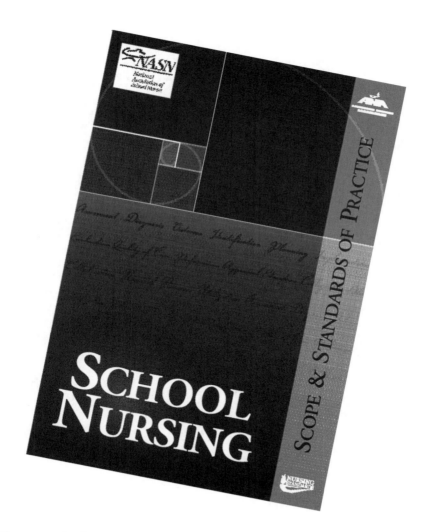

The content in this appendix is not current and is of historical significance only.

This appendix is not current and is of historical significance only.

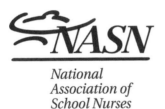

National
Association of
School Nurses

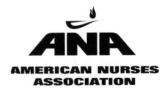

SCHOOL NURSING:

SCOPE AND STANDARDS

OF PRACTICE

AMERICAN NURSES ASSOCIATION
SILVER SPRING, MD
2005

This appendix is not current and is of historical significance only.

Library of Congress Cataloging-in-Publication data

National Association of School Nurses (U.S.)
 School nursing : scope and standards of practice / National Association of School Nurses.
  p. ; cm.
 Includes bibliographical references and index.
 ISBN-13: 978-1-55810-227-9
 ISBN-10: 1-55810-227-2
 1. School nursing—Standards—United States.
 [DNLM: 1. School Nursing.   2. Nursing Process. WY 113 N277sh 2005]   I. American Nurses Association.   II. Title.

RJ247.N38 2005
371.7'12—dc22   2005014707

The American Nurses Association (ANA) is a national professional association. This ANA publication—*School Nursing: Scope and Standards of Practice*—reflects the thinking of the nursing profession on various issues and should be reviewed in conjunction with state board of nursing policies and practices. State law, rules, and regulations govern the practice of nursing, while *School Nursing: Scope and Standards of Practice* guides nurses in the application of their professional skills and responsibilities.

Published by nursesbooks.org
The Publishing Program of ANA

American Nurses Association
8515 Georgia Avenue, Suite 400
Silver Spring, MD 20910
1-800-274-4ANA
http://www.nursingworld.org/

ANA is the only full-service professional organization representing the nation's 2.7 million Registered Nurses through its 54 constituent member associations. ANA advances the nursing profession by fostering high standards of nursing practice, promoting the economic and general welfare of nurses in the workplace, projecting a positive and realistic view of nursing, and lobbying the Congress and regulatory agencies on healthcare issues affecting nurses and the public.

The National Association of School Nurses is the leading worldwide expert for school health services and is the only organization that represents school nurses and school nursing interests exclusively. Its mission is to advance the delivery of professional school health services in order to promote optimal health and learning in students, primarily through its programs and resources for its members, advocacy and public relations activities, and research support and initiatives.

ISBN 978-1-55810-228-6   05SSSN   5M   06/05

First printing June 2005.

This appendix is not current and is of historical significance only.

CONTENTS

This appendix is not current and is of historical significance only.

This appendix is not current and is of historical significance only.

ACKNOWLEDGMENTS

The National Association of School Nurses wishes to acknowledge and thank the following organizational representatives who served on a task force to review the 2001 *Scope and Standards of Professional School Nursing Practice* and suggest revisions:

Roberta Bavin, MN, CPNP, CS
National Association of Pediatric Nurses and Practitioners

Julia Muennich Cowell, PhD, RNC, FAAN
American Public Health Association

Charlotte Burt, MSN, MA, RNBC, FASHA
American School Health Association

Linda Davis-Aldritt, RN, MA, PHN
National Association of State School Nurse Consultants

Maria Klein-Rivera, RNC, MSN
National Center for School Health Nursing

The National Association of School Nurses appreciates the work of the Board of Directors on this document and the following individuals for their expertise and contributions:

Carol Boal, BGS, RN, NCSN
NASN Executive Committee, Board of Directors, Wyoming

Sandi Delack, BSN, MEd, RN, CSNT
NASN Executive Committee, Board of Directors, Rhode Island

Cynthia Galemore, BSN, MSEd, RN, NCSN
NASN Executive Committee, Kansas

Janis Hootman, RN, PhD, NCSN
NASN President, Oregon

Sally Hrymak Hunter, RN, BSN, NCSN
NASN Vice President, New Mexico

Patricia Krin, MSN, APRN, FNP, NCSN
NASN Executive Committee, Connecticut

Wanda Miller, RN, MA, NCSN, FNASN
NASN Former President and Executive Director, Colorado

This appendix is not current and is of historical significance only.

Norma Nikkola, RN, BS, MS
NASN Board, Ohio

Susan Praeger, RN, EdD
School Nurse Educator, Ohio

Susanne Tullos, RN, MNSc, MSBA, NCSN
NASN Secretary, Arkansas

Susan Will, RN, MPH, NCSN, FNASN
NASN President-elect, Minnesota

Linda C. Wolfe, RN, BSN, MEd, NCSN
NASN Past President, Delaware

In addition, I wish to thank Dr. Carol Bickford, Senior Policy Fellow of the Department of Nursing Practice and Policy of the American Nurses Association, for her many suggestions and unfailing support during the review and revision process.

Elizabeth L. Thomas, RN, BS, MEd, NCSN
NASN Task Force Leader and Editor, Delaware

ANA Staff

Carol J. Bickford, PhD, RN,BC – Content editor
Yvonne Humes, MSA – Project coordinator
Winifred Carson, JD – Legal counsel

This appendix is not current and is of historical significance only.

PREFACE

The contents of this document have evolved over time to frame the current role and practice of school nurses in many locales across the country and in American schools abroad. School nursing has had standards of practice since 1983, when a task force of the National Association of School Nurses, chaired by Georgia McDonough of Arizona, produced the first set of standards specific to the specialty (ANA 1983). These were modeled on early generic standards authored by the American Nurses Association (ANA). The 1983 standards served school nursing well and were the basis for the development of three implementation manuals: one by the American School Health Association (Snyder 1991), and two by the National Association of School Nurses (Proctor 1990; Proctor, Lordi, and Zaiger 1993).

The scope of practice statement describes the who, what, where, when, why, and how of school nursing practice. Review and discussion by professional school nurses focused on answering these questions and resulted in the revised scope statement. Originally written by Leslie Cooper, RN, MSN, CS, FNP, and Donna Mazyck, RN, MS, NCSN, and first published with the standards in 2001, the Scope of Practice statement has been updated and expanded, but its character remains unchanged. The standards in this document are based on the template language in *Nursing: Scope and Standards of Practice* (ANA 2004). Careful additions and substitutions make this document unique to school nursing.

The scope and standards for school nursing were approved by the National Association of School Nurses Board of Directors in November 2004 and submitted to ANA's Committee on Nursing Practice Standards and Guidelines for review. In March 2005 the ANA Congress on Nursing Practice and Economics completed its review and approved the scope of practice statement for school nursing and acknowledged the standards of practice for school nursing.

Together, the scope statement and standards describe the professional expectations of school nurses. The standards serve as a definitive guide for role implementation, interpretation, and evaluation. They are useful for the writing of position descriptions for the school nurse and for planning relevant professional development programs. The scope

This appendix is not current and is of historical significance only.

and standards of school nursing practice are also used in conjunction with state nurse practice acts and other relevant laws or regulations to determine the adequacy of school nursing practice. This document further defines and clarifies the role of school nurses within schools and communities.

Dr. Janis Hootman, President of the National Association of School Nurses, often has spoken of the legacy that school nurses provide for their colleagues and clients. It is with great optimism that this framework is offered to school nurses to help them channel their vast energies into health and academic achievement for all students. The legacy of high expectations for a long healthy life and lifelong learning is a gift school nurses strive to give every day to their clients.

This appendix is not current and is of historical significance only.

INTRODUCTION

The Standards of School Nursing Practice and their accompanying measurement criteria describe and measure a competent level of school nursing practice and professional performance. Built on ANA's *Nursing: Scope and Standards of Practice* (ANA 2004) for registered nurses, these standards are authoritative statements of the accountability, direction, and evaluation of individuals in this specialty nursing practice. Composed of two sets—the Standards of Practice and the Standards of Professional Performance—these standards define how outcomes for school nurse activities can be measured.

The Standards of Practice reflect the six steps of the nursing process (assessment, diagnosis, outcomes identification, implementation, planning, and evaluation), which is the foundation for the critical thinking of all registered nurses. The Standards of Professional Performance describe the expected behaviors expected of the nurse in the role of a school nurse.

Also included in this book is a detailed statement on the scope of school nursing practice. This discussion describes the context of this specialty practice, effectively answering the essential questions: the who, what, where, when, why, and how of school nursing practice.

Current nursing practice reflects a number of themes that underlie all nursing practice and have significant meaning for school nursing practice (ANA 2004):

- Providing age-appropriate and culturally and ethnically sensitive care
- Maintaining a safe environment
- Educating patients [clients] about healthy practices and treatment modalities
- Assuring continuity of care
- Coordinating the care across settings and among caregivers
- Managing information
- Communicating effectively
- Utilizing technology.

This appendix is not current and is of historical significance only.

School nursing practice embraces and uses these themes in current practice. In fact, a communication standard was part of the *Scope and Standards of Professional School Nursing Practice* (NASN 2001). It is not a separate standard in the current publication because communication is part of each of the standards. Effective communication is still the cornerstone of the school nurse's practice.

Taken together, the contents of this book delineate the professional responsibilities of all school nurses engaged in clinical practice. This and other documents, such as position statements and issue briefs, could serve as the basis for:

- Quality improvement systems;
- Databases;
- Regulatory systems;
- Healthcare reimbursement and financial methodologies;
- Development and evaluation of nursing service delivery systems and organizational structures;
- Certification activities;
- Position descriptions and performance appraisals;
- Agency policies, procedures, and protocols; and
- Educational offerings.

Standards and practice guidelines must be evaluated regularly. School nurses are invited to provide feedback to the National Association of School Nurses regarding the usefulness, effectiveness, and comprehensiveness of this document. Keep in mind that it cannot account for all possible developments in practice. Guidelines, documents, and local protocols and procedures, as well as federal and state regulations and nurse practice acts, provide further direction.

This appendix is not current and is of historical significance only.

STANDARDS OF SCHOOL NURSING PRACTICE:
STANDARDS OF PRACTICE

STANDARD 1. ASSESSMENT
The school nurse collects comprehensive data pertinent to the client's health or the situation.

STANDARD 2. DIAGNOSIS
The school nurse analyzes the assessment data to determine the diagnosis or issues.

STANDARD 3. OUTCOMES IDENTIFICATION
The school nurse identifies expected outcomes for a plan individualized to the client or the situation.

STANDARD 4. PLANNING
The school nurse develops a plan that prescribes strategies and alternatives to attain expected outcomes.

STANDARD 5. IMPLEMENTATION
The school nurse implements the identified plan.

STANDARD 5A: COORDINATION OF CARE
The school nurse coordinates care delivery.

STANDARD 5B: HEALTH TEACHING AND HEALTH PROMOTION
The school nurse provides health education and employs strategies to promote health and a safe environment.

STANDARD 5C: CONSULTATION
The school nurse provides consultation to influence the identified plan, enhance the abilities of others, and effect change.

STANDARD 5D: PRESCRIPTIVE AUTHORITY AND TREATMENT
The advanced practice registered nurse uses prescriptive authority, procedures, referrals, treatments, and therapies in accordance with state and federal laws and regulations.

STANDARD 6. EVALUATION
The school nurse evaluates progress towards achievement of outcomes.

This appendix is not current and is of historical significance only.

STANDARDS OF SCHOOL NURSING PRACTICE:
STANDARDS OF PROFESSIONAL PERFORMANCE

STANDARD 7. QUALITY OF PRACTICE
The school nurse systematically enhances the quality and effectiveness of nursing practice.

STANDARD 8. EDUCATION
The school nurse attains knowledge and competency that reflects current school nursing practice.

STANDARD 9. PROFESSIONAL PRACTICE EVALUATION
The school nurse evaluates one's own nursing practice in relation to professional standards and guidelines, relevant statutes, rules, and regulations.

STANDARD 10. COLLEGIALITY
The school nurse interacts with, and contributes to the professional development of, peers and school personnel as colleagues.

STANDARD 11. COLLABORATION
The school nurse collaborates with the client, the family, school staff, and others in the conduct of school nursing practice.

STANDARD 12. ETHICS
The school nurse integrates ethical provisions in all areas of practice.

STANDARD 13. RESEARCH
The school nurse integrates research findings into practice.

STANDARD 14. RESOURCE UTILIZATION
The school nurse considers factors related to safety, effectiveness, cost, and impact on practice in the planning and delivery of school nursing services.

STANDARD 15. LEADERSHIP
The school nurse provides leadership in the professional practice setting and the profession.

STANDARD 16. PROGRAM MANAGEMENT
The school nurse manages school health services.

This appendix is not current and is of historical significance only.

SCOPE OF SCHOOL NURSING PRACTICE

Definitions and Distinguishing Characteristics

Nursing is the protection, promotion, and optimization of health and abilities, prevention of illness and injury, alleviation of suffering through the diagnosis and treatment of human response, and advocacy in the care of individuals, families, communities, and populations (ANA 2003a). "School Nursing is a specialized practice of professional nursing that advances the well-being, academic success, and lifelong achievement and health of students. To that end, school nurses facilitate positive student responses to normal development; promote health and safety; intervene with actual and potential health problems; provide case management services; and actively collaborate with others to build student and family capacity for adaptation, self-management, self advocacy, and learning" (NASN 1999b).

School nursing takes place primarily within local education agencies serving school-age children. However, school nurses also provide services in alternative sites (e.g., juvenile justice centers, alternative treatment centers, preschools, college campuses, learning sites for children of personnel in the armed services, and residential campuses) and within the larger surrounding community, at students' homes, vocational/occupational settings, environmental camps, field trips, school-sanctioned competitions, and sporting events.

The school nurse is likely to be the only healthcare provider in the educational setting. Unlike other healthcare workers—such as occupational therapists, physical therapists, and school psychologists, all of whom have specific defined caseloads—the school nurse is responsible for all students in a given school, district, or region. The school nurse collaborates with other health professionals to provide successful interventions for positive client outcomes. School nurses are frequently called upon to delegate nursing care to teachers, school office staff, classroom assistants, and other unlicensed assistive personnel (UAP). School nurses must be fully aware of the applicable laws, regulations, and standards pertaining to delegation of nursing tasks to others. Some states have laws or regulations prohibiting such delegation.

This appendix is not current and is of historical significance only.

School nurses are most commonly employed by local school districts or education systems, although health systems such as public health, hospitals, and private health corporations may be the employer. School nurses work in a variety of delivery models such as consultant or direct services provider. They work with individuals, as well as populations, serving students from birth through age 21 or even older. The "client" of the school nurse includes not only the student, but also the student's family, the staff and faculty of the school, and the school community at large. Key roles of the school nurse include clinician, advocate, social service coordinator, health educator, liaison, and interdisciplinary student services team member (Wolfe 2005):

> Since the inception of school nursing, at the turn of the twentieth century, the specialty practice has embraced both health and education initiatives to promote the health and well-being of children. Lillian Wald, founder, envisioned a role for the school nurse to serve all, regardless of economic or social stature, or origin of nationality. She merged public health goals (to be free of communicable disease, which was of epidemic proportions), educational goals (to eliminate absenteeism from exclusion based upon contagious status), and social goals (to build literate and productive citizens). Medical goals focused on identification and exclusion of children. School nursing goals focused on inclusion.

In today's world, communicable diseases are not the only health related barriers to education. Some of the issues school nurses must address include:

- Child abuse and neglect;
- Domestic and school violence;
- Child and adolescent obesity and inactivity;
- Suicide;
- Alcohol, tobacco, and other drug use;
- Adolescent pregnancy and parenting;
- Environmental health;
- Physical and emotional disabilities and their consequences;
- Mental health;

This appendix is not current and is of historical significance only.

- Children with complex physical needs; and

- Lack of health insurance coverage

School nursing is the pivotal component in continuity of care through the coordination, planning, delivery, and assessment of school health services. School nurses use the nursing process, the six steps of which—assessment, diagnosis, outcomes identification, implementation, planning, evaluation—and are the basis for the Standards of Practice. Among its other uses, this process helps to promote student and staff health and safety. School nurses also develop team relationships within the school and with community providers so that care is coordinated across settings to meet individual health needs and to avoid duplication of services.

The school nurse's primary role is to support student learning by acting as an advocate and liaison between the home, the school, and the medical community regarding concerns that may affect a student's ability to learn (NASN 1999b). Specific responsibilities are as diverse as the clients and communities served. The school nurse provides comprehensive services in all components of a coordinated school health program (Marx, Wooley, and Northrup 1998):

- Health services—Serves as the coordinator of the health services program, provides nursing care, advocates for health rights and optimization of health and abilities, and provides referral for services.

- Health education—Provides appropriate health information that promotes health and informed healthcare decisions, prevents disease, and enhances school performance.

- Environment—Identifies health and safety concerns in the school community, promotes a safe and nurturing school environment, and promotes injury prevention.

- Nutrition—Supports school food service programs and promotes the benefits of healthy eating patterns.

- Physical education and activity—Promotes healthy activities, physical education, and sports policies and practices that promote safety, good sportsmanship, and a lifelong active lifestyle.

- Counseling and mental health—Provides health counseling, assesses mental health needs, provides interventions, refers students to appropriate school staff or community agencies, and provides follow-up once treatment is prescribed.

This appendix is not current and is of historical significance only.

- Parent and community involvement—Promotes community participation in assuring a healthy school and serves as school liaison to a health advisory committee.

- Staff wellness—Provides health education and counseling, and promotes healthy activities and environment for school staff.

Continuum of School Nursing Practice

School nursing exists on a continuum from the beginner through the veteran. Both the generalist school nurse and the school nurse practitioner with advanced practice training must hold current licensure as registered nurses in the state in which they practice.

Because of the complexity of issues addressed by the school nurse, the National Association of School Nurses (NASN) recommends as the minimum education for a school nurse a baccalaureate degree in nursing (BSN) from an accredited college or university, as well as state certification in states that require or recommend certification for state school nurses. Those school nurse generalists who have not acquired these credentials are strongly encouraged to aspire to and achieve these qualifications. NASN also recommends that school nurse generalists demonstrate their knowledge of school nursing by acquiring certification in the specialty of school nursing, which also requires a bachelor's degree. The NCSN credential is awarded by the National Board for Certification of School Nurses to those who pass the school nurse certification examination.

The continuum of school nurse practice includes other school nurse professionals such as advanced practice registered nurses, school nurse consultants, school nurse supervisors and administrators, lead nurses, or team leaders. There are school nurses in lead roles at school districts, regions, counties, and at the state level. As lifelong learners, school nurses seek professional development to increase critical thinking skills and professional judgment as well as to maintain current skills and knowledge. In some states, professional development is tied to licensure, but, in any case, school nurses have a professional responsibility to increase their own personal body of knowledge.

School nurses, whether generalists or advanced practice nurses, employ a community health focus in their practice. Health services are provided within the framework of primary, secondary, and tertiary pre-

This appendix is not current and is of historical significance only.

vention. Programs and services are offered with the goal of prevention—to individual students as well as to the entire school community.

School Nurse

The school nurse provides health education, health promotion, preventive health services, health assessment, and referral services to clients and staff. The actions of the school nurse focus on strengthening and facilitating students' educational outcomes, and may be directed toward individual students, family, segments of the school population, the entire school population, the school community, or the larger surrounding community. The school nurse serves as the liaison between the school, community healthcare providers, and the school-based or school-linked clinics. "As the healthcare expert within the school system, the school nurse takes a leadership role in the development and evaluation of school health policies. The school nurse participates in and provides leadership to coordinated school health programs, crisis/disaster management teams, and school health advisory councils" (NASN 2002).

The school nurse must demonstrate expertise in pediatric and adolescent health assessment, community health, and adult and child mental health nursing. Strong skills in health promotion, assessment and referral, communication, leadership, organization, and time management are essential. Knowledge of health and education laws that affect students is critical, as are teaching strategies for the delivery of health education to clients and staff, individually and collectively. School nurses are often physically isolated from other nursing and healthcare colleagues; therefore they need to be comfortable and skilled with independent management of the health office and the client caseload (Wolfe 2005).

The functions of the school nurse are to promote academic success and provide optimal nursing care to the entire school community. To these ends, the school nurse most often employs the six steps of the nursing process (adapted from ANA 2004):

- Assessment—Collects comprehensive data.

- Diagnosis—Analyzes data to determine the *nursing* diagnoses or issues.

- Outcomes identification—Identifies *measurable* expected outcomes for a plan.

This appendix is not current and is of historical significance only.

- Planning—Develops a plan to attain expected outcomes.
- Implementation—Implements the plan.
- Evaluation—Evaluates progress toward attainment of outcomes.

Advanced Practice Registered Nurse

Some school nurses may meet the standards for Advanced Practice Registered Nurses (APRNs) as a result of their education, experience, skill, and authority to practice by their state licensing board. APRNs have advanced degrees and national certification in their specialty. They can be nurse practitioners or clinical specialists or both. They are differentiated by educational preparation and clinical practice. APRNs are often part of an enhanced school services team that offers health care beyond basic core services. The APRN working in the school must be knowledgeable about and competent in the standards expected of the school nurse. APRNs can offer a cost-effective solution to identified needs for students who do not receive "consistent, appropriate medical care" contributing to barriers to learning. "The anticipated outcome is more health needs of students being met, resulting in a positive impact on the health and educational performance of students" (NASN 2003).

Nursing Role Specialty

Nursing role specialties are advanced levels of nursing practice that intersect with other bodies of knowledge, have a direct influence on nursing practice, and support the delivery of direct care rendered to patients by other registered nurses. School nurses with additional professional experience and education may elect to conduct their school nursing practice within administration, education, case management, informatics, research, or other role specialties. The school nurse in a nursing role specialty should have a master's or doctoral degree. The school nurse in a role specialty is expected to comply with the standards of practice and professional performance and the associated measurement criteria for all school nurses and the additional measurement criteria for the role specialist. Other resources, such as *Scope and Standards for Nurse Administrators* (ANA 2003b), may provide additional direction.

This appendix is not current and is of historical significance only.

Ethical Considerations

The degree to which the school environment supports nursing practice affects the delivery of nursing care. *Healthy People 2010* cites a recommended school nurse to student ratio of 1:750 in the national health objectives (USDHHS 2000). The appropriateness of this ratio is dependent on the needs of the school population. School nurses must be able to practice nursing in an educationally focused system and clearly communicate in both the healthcare and education arenas. School nurses face unique policy, funding, and supervisory issues.

The school nurse practices in an environment that has changed dramatically since the early twentieth century. The Individuals with Disabilities Act of 1997, section 504 of the Rehabilitation Act of 1973, and the Americans with Disabilities Act of 1990 removed barriers that hindered students' access to education. Education regulations heighten the complexity of decision-making and practice, such as those of the Family Education Rights and Privacy Act (FERPA) of 1974, and subsequent amendments regarding Do Not Resuscitate orders in the school setting. The restrictions to medical information imposed by the Health Information Portability and Accessibility Act (HIPAA) of 1996 present an ongoing challenge to the school nurse who needs information about student medical needs for adequate care at school.

School nurses are advocates for their clients—students, families, school staff, and the community. They provide care to their clients that is both age-appropriate and culturally and ethnically sensitive. School nurses promote active informed participation in health decisions. They respect the individual's right to be treated with dignity, and understand the ethical and legal issues surrounding an individual's right to privacy and confidentiality. The school nurse treats all members of the school community equally, regardless of race, gender, social or economic status, culture, age, sexual orientation, disability, or religion.

The school nurse maintains the highest level of competency by enhancing professional knowledge and skills, collaborating with peers and other health professionals and community agencies, and adhering to these documents: *Nursing's Social Policy Statement* (ANA 2003a), *Code of Ethics for Nurses with Interpretive Statements* (ANA 2001), *Code of Ethics with Interpretive Statements for the School Nurse* (NASN 1999a), and the current scope and standards of school nursing. School nurses participate

This appendix is not current and is of historical significance only.

in the profession's efforts to advance the standards of practice, expand the body of knowledge through nursing research, and improve conditions of employment. School nurses are expected to regulate themselves; they are responsible to themselves and others for the quality of their practice. The school nurse is autonomous and must engage in considerable reflection for quality assurance.

Summary

School nurses continue to adapt their practice to a changing world. New challenges continue to present themselves, as do new tools to assist the school nurse in meeting these challenges. As technology advances, so does the school nurse's practice. Students with more complex daily health needs, as well as those requiring intermittent on-site medical treatments, are in schools across America every day. Technology is available, not only as a classroom tool and for expanded school health record keeping, but also to give students with health impairments greater access to the education to which they are entitled.

Healthy children are successful learners. The school nurse has a multifaceted role within the school setting, one that supports the physical, emotional, mental, and social health of students and their success in the learning process (NASN 2002). The future of school nursing rests on the ability of the school nurse to successfully meet the challenges in the health and education communities.

This appendix is not current and is of historical significance only.

STANDARDS OF SCHOOL NURSING PRACTICE
STANDARDS OF PRACTICE

School Nursing is a specialized practice of professional nursing that advances the well-being, academic success, and lifelong achievement and health of students. To that end, school nurses facilitate positive student responses to normal development; promote health and safety; intervene with actual and potential health problems; provide case management services; and actively collaborate with others to build student and family capacity for adaptation, self-management, self-advocacy, and learning. (NASN 1999b)

STANDARD 1. ASSESSMENT
The school nurse collects comprehensive data pertinent to the client's* health or the situation.

Measurement Criteria:

The school nurse:

- Systematically compares and contrasts clinical findings with normal and abnormal variations and developmental events in forming a nursing diagnosis.

- Involves the client, family, school staff, other healthcare providers, and school community, as appropriate, in holistic data collection.

- Prioritizes data collection activities based on the client's immediate condition, or anticipated needs of the client or situation.

- Uses appropriate evidence-based assessment techniques and instruments in collecting pertinent data.

- Uses analytical models and problem-solving tools.

---

* Client is used in these standards to better reflect the diversity of the recipients of school nursing practice. The client can be a student, the student and family as a unit, the school population, or the school community, including faculty and staff. The focus of care may shift from individual needs to the needs of a group.

Continued ▶

This appendix is not current and is of historical significance only.

- Synthesizes available data, information, and knowledge relevant to the situation to identify patterns and variances.
- Documents relevant data in a retrievable format.

Additional Measurement Criterion for the Advanced Practice Registered Nurse:

The advanced practice registered nurse:

- Initiates and interprets diagnostic tests and procedures relevant to the client's current status.

This appendix is not current and is of historical significance only.

STANDARD 2. DIAGNOSIS
The school nurse analyzes the assessment data to determine the diagnoses or issues.

Measurement Criteria:

The school nurse:

- Derives the nursing diagnoses or issues based on assessment data.

- Validates the nursing diagnoses or issues with the client, family, school staff, school community, and other healthcare providers when possible and appropriate.

- Documents nursing diagnoses or issues in a manner that facilitates the determination of the expected outcomes and plan.

- Uses standardized language or recognized terminology to document the nursing diagnosis in a retrievable form.

Additional Measurement Criteria for the Advanced Practice Registered Nurse:

The advanced practice registered nurse:

- Systematically compares and contrasts clinical findings with normal and abnormal variations and developmental events in formulating a differential diagnosis.

- Utilizes complex data and information obtained during interview, examination, and diagnostic procedures in identifying diagnoses.

- Assists staff in developing and maintaining competency in the diagnostic process.

This appendix is not current and is of historical significance only.

STANDARD 3. OUTCOMES IDENTIFICATION
The school nurse identifies expected outcomes for a plan individualized to the client or the situation.

Measurement Criteria:

The school nurse:

- Involves the client, family, school staff, and other healthcare providers in formulating expected outcomes when possible and appropriate.

- Derives culturally appropriate expected outcomes from the diagnoses.

- Considers associated risks, benefits, costs, current scientific evidence, and clinical expertise when formulating expected outcomes.

- Defines expected outcomes in terms of the client, client values, ethical considerations, environment, or situation with such consideration as associated risks, benefits and costs, and current scientific evidence.

- Includes a time estimate for attainment of expected outcomes.

- Develops expected outcomes that provide direction for continuity of care.

- Modifies expected outcomes based on changes in the status of the client or evaluation of the situation.

- Documents expected outcomes as measurable goals.

- Uses standardized language or recognized terminology to document the outcome in a retrievable form.

Additional Measurement Criteria for the Advanced Practice Registered Nurse:

The advanced practice registered nurse:

- Identifies expected outcomes that incorporate scientific evidence and are achievable through implementation of evidence-based practices.

This appendix is not current and is of historical significance only.

- Identifies expected outcomes that incorporate cost and clinical effectiveness, client satisfaction, and continuity and consistency among providers.
- Supports the use of clinical guidelines linked to positive client outcomes.

This appendix is not current and is of historical significance only.

STANDARD 4. PLANNING
The school nurse develops a plan that prescribes strategies and alternatives to attain expected outcomes.

Measurement Criteria:

The school nurse:

- Develops an individualized healthcare plan considering the client characteristics or the situation (e.g., age and culturally appropriate, environmentally sensitive), with appropriate strategies for health promotion and disease prevention.

- Develops the plan in conjunction with the client, family, school community, and others, as appropriate.

- Creates individual healthcare plans as a component of the program for clients with special healthcare needs.

- Provides for continuity within the plan.

- Incorporates an implementation pathway or timeline within the plan.

- Establishes the plan priorities with the client, family, school community, and others as appropriate.

- Utilizes the plan to provide direction to other members of the school team.

- Defines the plan to reflect current statutes, rules and regulations, and standards.

- Integrates current trends and research affecting care in the planning process.

- Considers the economic impact of the plan.

- Uses standardized language or recognized terminology to document the plan in a retrievable form.

Additional Measurement Criteria for the Advanced Practice Registered Nurse:

The advanced practice registered nurse:

- Identifies assessment, diagnostic strategies, and therapeutic interventions within the plan that reflect current evidence, including data, research, literature, and expert clinical knowledge.

This appendix is not current and is of historical significance only.

- Selects or designs strategies to meet the multifaceted needs of complex clients.

- Includes the synthesis of client's values and beliefs regarding nursing and medical therapies within the plan.

Additional Measurement Criteria for the Nursing Role Specialty:

The school nurse in a nursing role specialty:

- Participates in the design and development of multidisciplinary and interdisciplinary processes to address the situation or issue.

- Contributes to the development and continuous improvement of organizational systems that support the planning process.

- Supports the integration of clinical, human, and financial resources to enhance and complete the decision-making processes.

This appendix is not current and is of historical significance only.

STANDARD 5. IMPLEMENTATION
The school nurse implements the identified plan.

Measurement Criteria:

The school nurse:

- Implements the plan in a safe and timely manner.
- Documents implementation and any modifications, including changes or omissions, of the specified plan.
- Utilizes evidence-based interventions and treatments specific to the diagnosis or problem.
- Utilizes community resources and systems to implement the plan.
- Collaborates with nursing colleagues and others to implement the plan.
- Provides interventions in compliance with these standards of practice and professional performance.
- Uses standardized language or recognized terminology to document implementation of the plan in a retrievable form.

Additional Measurement Criteria for the Advanced Practice Registered Nurse:

The advanced practice registered nurse:

- Facilitates utilization of systems and community resources to implement the plan.
- Supports collaboration with school nursing colleagues and other nursing colleagues and disciplines to implement the plan.
- Incorporates new knowledge and strategies to initiate change in school nursing care practices if desired outcomes are not achieved.

Additional Measurement Criteria for the Nursing Role Specialty:

The school nurse in a nursing role specialty:

- Implements the plan using principles and concepts of project or systems management.
- Fosters organizational systems that support implementation of the plan.

This appendix is not current and is of historical significance only.

STANDARD 5A: COORDINATION OF CARE
The school nurse coordinates care delivery.

Measurement Criteria:

The school nurse:

- Coordinates creation and implementation of the individual health-care plan.
- Documents the coordination of the care.

Measurement Criteria for the Advanced Practice Registered Nurse:

The advanced practice registered nurse:

- Provides leadership in the coordination of multidisciplinary health care for integrated delivery of client care services.
- Synthesizes data and information to prescribe necessary education and healthcare system and community support measures, including environmental modifications.
- Coordinates education and healthcare system and community resources that enhance delivery of care across continuums.

This appendix is not current and is of historical significance only.

STANDARD 5B: HEALTH TEACHING AND HEALTH PROMOTION
The school nurse provides health education and employs strategies to promote health and a safe environment.

Measurement Criteria:

The school nurse:

- Provides general health education to the student body at large through direct classroom instruction or expert consultation.

- Provides health teaching that addresses such topics as healthy lifestyles, risk-reducing behaviors, developmental needs, activities of daily living, and preventive self-care as appropriate to client developmental levels.

- Uses health promotion and health teaching methods appropriate to the situation and the client's developmental level, learning needs, readiness, ability to learn, language preference, and culture.

- Promotes self-care and safety through the education of the school community regarding health issues.*

- Promotes health principles through the coordinated school health program for all in the school community.

- Seeks opportunities for feedback and evaluation of the effectiveness of the strategies used.

- Participates in the assessment of needs for health education and health instruction for the school community.*

- Provides individual and group health teaching and counseling for and with clients.*

- Participates in the design and development of health education materials, and other health education activities.*

- Participates in the evaluation of health curricula and health instructional materials and activities.*

- Acts as a primary resource person to school staff (and others as appropriate) regarding health education and health education materials.*

---

*Adapted from Proctor, Lordi, and Zaiger 1993 and NASN and ANA 2001.

This appendix is not current and is of historical significance only.

Additional Measurement Criteria for the Advanced Practice Registered Nurse:

The advanced practice registered nurse:

- Synthesizes empirical evidence on risk behaviors, learning theories, behavioral change theories, motivational theories, epidemiology, and other related theories and frameworks when designing health information and client education.

- Designs health information and client education appropriate to the client's developmental level, learning needs, readiness to learn, and cultural values and beliefs.

- Evaluates health information resources, such as the Internet, within the area of practice for accuracy, readability, and comprehensibility to help client's access quality health information.

This appendix is not current and is of historical significance only.

STANDARD 5C: CONSULTATION

The school nurse provides consultation to influence the identified plan, enhance the abilities of others, and effect change.

Measurement Criteria:

The school nurse:

- Synthesizes data, information, theoretical frameworks, and evidence when providing consultation.

- Facilitates the effectiveness of a consultation by involving the stakeholders in the decision-making process.

- Communicates consultation recommendations that influence the identified plan, facilitate understanding by involved stakeholders, enhance the work of others, and effect change.

Measurement Criteria for the Advanced Practice Registered Nurse:

The advanced practice registered nurse:

- Synthesizes clinical data, theoretical frameworks, and evidence when providing consultation.

- Facilitates the effectiveness of a consultation by involving the client when appropriate in decision-making and negotiating role responsibilities.

- Communicates consultation recommendations that facilitate change.

This appendix is not current and is of historical significance only.

STANDARD 5D: PRESCRIPTIVE AUTHORITY AND TREATMENT
The advanced practice registered nurse uses prescriptive authority, procedures, referrals, treatments, and therapies in accordance with state and federal laws and regulations.

Measurement Criteria for the Advanced Practice Registered Nurse:

The advanced practice registered nurse:

- Prescribes evidence-based treatments, therapies, and procedures considering the client's comprehensive healthcare needs.

- Prescribes pharmacologic agents based on a current knowledge of pharmacology and physiology.

- Prescribes specific pharmacological agents and/or treatments based on clinical indicators, the client's status and needs, and the results of diagnostic and laboratory tests.

- Evaluates therapeutic and potential adverse effects of pharmacological and non-pharmacological treatments.

- Provides client and family with information about intended effects and potential adverse effects of proposed prescriptive therapies.

- Provides information about costs, and alternative treatments and procedures, as appropriate.

This appendix is not current and is of historical significance only.

STANDARD 6. EVALUATION
The school nurse evaluates progress towards attainment of outcomes.

Measurement Criteria:

The school nurse:

- Conducts a systematic, ongoing, and criterion-based evaluation of the outcomes in relation to the structures and processes prescribed by the plan and the indicated timeline.

- Includes the client and others involved in the care or situation in the evaluative process.

- Evaluates the effectiveness of the planned strategies in relation to client responses and the attainment of the expected outcomes.

- Documents the results of the evaluation.

- Uses ongoing assessment data to revise the diagnoses, the outcomes, the plan, and the implementation as needed.

- Disseminates the results to the client and others involved in the care or situation, as appropriate, in accordance with client and parent directions, and state and federal laws and regulations.

Additional Measurement Criteria for the Advanced Practice Registered Nurse:

The advanced practice registered nurse:

- Evaluates the accuracy of the diagnosis and effectiveness of the interventions in relationship to the patient's attainment of expected outcomes.

- Synthesizes the results of the evaluation analyses to determine the impact of the plan on the affected clients, families, groups, communities, and institutions.

- Uses the results of the evaluation analyses to make or recommend process or structural changes, including policy, procedure, or protocol documentation, as appropriate.

This appendix is not current and is of historical significance only.

Additional Measurement Criteria for the Nursing Role Specialty:

The school nurse in a nursing role specialty:

- Uses the results of the evaluation analyses to make or recommend process or structural changes, including policy, procedure, or protocol documentation, as appropriate.

- Synthesizes the results of the evaluation analyses to determine the impact of the plan on the affected clients, families, groups, school communities, and institutions, networks, and organizations.

This appendix is not current and is of historical significance only.

STANDARDS OF PROFESSIONAL PERFORMANCE

STANDARD 7. QUALITY OF PRACTICE
The school nurse systematically enhances the quality and effectiveness of nursing practice.

Measurement Criteria:

The school nurse:

- Demonstrates quality by documenting the application of the nursing process in a responsible, accountable, and ethical manner.
- Uses the results of quality improvement activities to initiate changes in school nursing practice and in the healthcare delivery system.
- Uses creativity and innovation in school nursing practice to improve care delivery.
- Incorporates new knowledge to initiate changes in school nursing practice if desired outcomes are not achieved.
- Participates in quality improvement activities. Such activities may include:
  - Identifying aspects of practice important for quality monitoring.
  - Using indicators developed to monitor quality and effectiveness of nursing practice.
  - Collecting data to monitor quality and effectiveness of school nursing practice.
  - Analyzing quality data to identify opportunities for improving school nursing practice.
  - Formulating recommendations to improve school nursing practice or outcomes.
  - Implementing activities to enhance the quality of school nursing practice.

Continued ▶

This appendix is not current and is of historical significance only.

- Developing, implementing, and evaluating policies, procedures and/or guidelines to improve the quality of school nursing practice.

- Participating on interdisciplinary teams to evaluate clinical care or health services.

- Participating in efforts to minimize costs and unnecessary duplication.

- Analyzing factors related to safety, satisfaction, effectiveness, and cost–benefit options.

- Analyzing organizational systems for barriers.

- Obtaining and maintaining national certification in school nursing as well as state certification (if available).

- Implementing processes to remove or decrease barriers within organizational systems.

Additional Measurement Criteria for the Advanced Practice Registered Nurse:

The advanced practice registered nurse:

- Obtains and maintains professional certification if available in the area of expertise.

- Designs quality improvement initiatives.

- Implements initiatives to evaluate the need for change.

- Evaluates the practice environment and quality of nursing care rendered in relation to existing evidence, identifying opportunities for the generation and use of research.

Additional Measurement Criteria for the Nursing Role Specialty:

The school nurse in a nursing role specialty:

- Obtains and maintains professional certification if available in the area of expertise.

- Designs quality improvement initiatives.

- Implements initiatives to evaluate the need for change.

- Evaluates the practice environment in relation to existing evidence, identifying opportunities for the generation and use of research.

This appendix is not current and is of historical significance only.

STANDARD 8. EDUCATION
The school nurse attains knowledge and competency that reflects current school nursing practice.

Measurement Criteria:

The school nurse:

- Participates in ongoing educational activities related to appropriate knowledge bases and professional issues.

- Demonstrates a commitment to lifelong learning through self-reflection and inquiry to identify learning needs.

- Seeks experiences that reflect current practice in order to maintain skills and competence in clinical practice or role performance.

- Acquires knowledge and skills appropriate to the specialty area, practice setting, role, or situation.

- Maintains professional records that provide evidence of competency and lifelong learning.

- Seeks experiences and formal and independent learning activities to maintain and develop clinical and professional skills and knowledge.

Additional Measurement Criterion for the Advanced Practice Registered Nurse:

The advanced practice registered nurse:

- Uses current healthcare research findings and other evidence to expand clinical knowledge, enhance role performance, and increase knowledge of professional issues.

Additional Measurement Criterion for the Nursing Role Specialty:

The school nurse in a nursing role specialty:

- Uses current research findings and other evidence to expand knowledge, enhance role performance, and increase knowledge of professional issues.

This appendix is not current and is of historical significance only.

STANDARD 9. PROFESSIONAL PRACTICE EVALUATION
The school nurse evaluates one's own nursing practice in relation to professional practice standards and guidelines, relevant statutes, rules, and regulations.

Measurement Criteria:

- The school nurse's practice reflects the application of knowledge of current practice standards, guidelines, statutes, rules, and regulations.

- The school nurse:

  - Provides age-appropriate care in a culturally and ethnically sensitive manner.

  - Engages in self-evaluation of practice on a regular basis, identifying areas of strength as well as areas in which professional development would be beneficial.

  - Obtains informal feedback regarding one's own practice from clients, peers, professional colleagues, and others.

  - Participates in systematic peer review as appropriate.

  - Takes action to achieve goals identified during the evaluation process.

  - Provides rationales for practice beliefs, decisions, and actions as part of the informal and formal evaluation processes.

Additional Measurement Criterion for the Advanced Practice Registered Nurse:

The advanced practice registered nurse:

- Engages in a formal process seeking feedback regarding one's own practice from clients, peers, professional colleagues, and others.

Additional Measurement Criterion for the Nursing Role Specialty:

The school nurse in a nursing role specialty:

- Engages in a formal process seeking feedback regarding role performance from individuals, professional colleagues, representatives and administrators of corporate entities, and others.

This appendix is not current and is of historical significance only.

STANDARD 10. COLLEGIALITY
The school nurse interacts with, and contributes to the professional development of, peers and school personnel as colleagues.

Measurement Criteria:

The school nurse:

- Shares knowledge and skills with peers and colleagues as evidenced by such activities as multidisciplinary student assistance conferences or presentations at formal or informal meetings.

- Provides peers with feedback regarding their practice or role performance.

- Interacts with peers and colleagues to enhance one's own professional nursing practice and role performance and the health care of the school community.

- Maintains compassionate and caring relationships with peers and colleagues.

- Contributes to an environment that is conducive to the education of healthcare professionals and the whole school community.

- Contributes to a supportive and healthy work environment.

- Participates in appropriate professional organizations in a membership or leadership capacity.

Additional Measurement Criteria for the Advanced Practice Registered Nurse:

The advanced practice registered nurse:

- Models expert practice to interdisciplinary team members and healthcare consumers.

- Mentors other registered nurses and colleagues as appropriate.

- Participates with interdisciplinary teams that contribute to role development and advanced nursing practice and health care.

Continued ▶

This appendix is not current and is of historical significance only.

Additional Measurement Criteria for the Nursing Role Specialty:

The school nurse in a nursing role specialty:

- Participates on multi-professional teams that contribute to role development and, directly or indirectly, advance nursing practice and health services.

- Mentors other registered nurses and colleagues as appropriate.

This appendix is not current and is of historical significance only.

STANDARD 11. COLLABORATION
The school nurse collaborates with the client, the family, school staff, and others in the conduct of school nursing practice.

Measurement Criteria:

The school nurse:

- Communicates with the client, the family, and healthcare providers regarding client care and the school nurse's role in the delivery of that care.

- Collaborates in creating a documented healthcare plan that is focused on outcomes and decisions related to care and delivery of services and indicates communication with clients, families, and others.

- Partners with others to effect change and generate positive outcomes through knowledge of the client or situation.

- Documents referrals, including provisions for continuity of care.

Additional Measurement Criteria for the Advanced Practice Registered Nurse:

The advanced practice registered nurse:

- Partners with other disciplines to enhance patient care through interdisciplinary activities, such as education, consultation, management, technological development, or research opportunities.

- Facilitates an interdisciplinary process with other members of the healthcare team.

- Documents plan-of-care communications, rationales for plan-of-care changes, and collaborative discussions to improve patient care.

Additional Measurement Criteria for the Nursing Role Specialty:

The school nurse in a nursing role specialty:

- Partners with others to enhance health care, and ultimately client care, through interdisciplinary activities such as education, consultation, management, technological development, or research.

- Documents plans, communications, rationales for plan changes, and collaborative discussions.

This appendix is not current and is of historical significance only.

STANDARD 12. ETHICS
The school nurse integrates ethical provisions in all areas of practice.

Measurement Criteria:

The school nurse:

- Uses *Code of Ethics for Nurses with Interpretive Statements* (ANA 2001) and *Code of Ethics with Interpretive Statements for School Nurses* (NASN 1999a) to guide practice.

- Delivers care in a manner that preserves and protects client autonomy, dignity, and rights, sensitive to diversity in the school setting.

- Maintains client confidentiality within legal and regulatory parameters of both health and education.

- Serves as a client advocate assisting clients in developing skills for self-advocacy.

- Maintains a therapeutic and professional client–nurse relationship with appropriate professional role boundaries.

- Demonstrates a commitment to practicing self-care, managing stress, and connecting with self and others.

- Contributes to resolving ethical issues of clients, colleagues, or systems as evidenced in such activities as participating on ethics committees.

- Reports illegal, incompetent, or impaired practices.

- Seeks available resources to formulate ethical decisions.

Additional Measurement Criteria for the Advanced Practice Registered Nurse:

The advanced practice registered nurse:

- Informs the client of the risks, benefits, and outcomes of healthcare regimens.

- Participates in interdisciplinary teams that address ethical risks, benefits, and outcomes.

This appendix is not current and is of historical significance only.

Additional Measurement Criteria for the Nursing Role Specialty:

The school nurse in a nursing role specialty:

- Participates on multidisciplinary and interdisciplinary teams that address ethical risks, benefits, and outcomes.

- Informs administrators or others of the risks, benefits, and outcomes of programs and decisions that affect healthcare delivery.

This appendix is not current and is of historical significance only.

STANDARD 13. RESEARCH
The school nurse integrates research findings into practice.

Measurement Criteria:

The school nurse:

- Utilizes the best available evidence, including research findings, to guide practice decisions.

- Actively participates in research activities at various levels appropriate to the school nurse's education and position. Such activities may include:

  - Identifying clinical problems specific to nursing research (client care and nursing practice).

  - Participating in data collection (surveys, pilot projects, formal studies).

  - Participating in a formal committee or program.

  - Sharing research activities or findings with peers and others.

  - Conducting research.

  - Critically analyzing and interpreting research for application to practice.

  - Using research findings in the development of policies, procedures, and standards of practice in client care.

  - Incorporating research as a basis for learning.

  - Contributing to school nursing literature.

Additional Measurement Criteria for the Advanced Practice Registered Nurse:

The advanced practice registered nurse:

- Contributes to nursing knowledge by conducting or synthesizing research that discovers, examines, and evaluates knowledge, theories, criteria, and creative approaches to improve healthcare practice.

- Formally disseminates research findings through activities such as presentations, publications, consultation, and journal clubs.

This appendix is not current and is of historical significance only.

Additional Measurement Criteria for the Nursing Role Specialty:

The school nurse in a nursing role specialty:

- Contributes to nursing knowledge by conducting or synthesizing research that discovers, examines, and evaluates knowledge, theories, criteria, and creative approaches to improve health care.

- Formally disseminates research findings through activities such as presentations, publications, consultation, and journal clubs.

This appendix is not current and is of historical significance only.

STANDARD **14.** RESOURCE UTILIZATION
The school nurse considers factors related to safety, effectiveness, cost, and impact on practice in the planning and delivery of school nursing services.

Measurement Criteria:

The school nurse:

- Evaluates factors such as safety, effectiveness, availability, cost and benefits, efficiencies, and impact on practice, when choosing among practice options that would result in the same expected outcome.

- Assists the client and family in identifying and securing appropriate and available services to address health-related needs.

- Assigns or delegates tasks, based on the needs and condition of the client, potential for harm, stability of the client's condition, complexity of the task, and predictability of the outcome; as defined and permitted by individual state nurse practice acts; and according to the knowledge and skills of the designated caregiver.

- Assists the client and school community in becoming informed consumers about the options, costs, risks, and benefits of health promotion, health education, school health services, and individualized health interventions for clients.

Additional Measurement Criteria for the Advanced Practice Registered Nurse:

The advanced practice registered nurse:

- Utilizes organizational and community resources to formulate multidisciplinary or interdisciplinary plans of care.

- Develops innovative solutions for client care problems that address effective resource utilization and maintenance of quality.

- Develops evaluation strategies to demonstrate cost effectiveness, cost–benefit, and efficiency factors associated with nursing practice.

Additional Measurement Criteria for the Nursing Role Specialty:

The school nurse in a nursing role specialty:

- Develops innovative solutions and applies strategies to obtain appropriate resources for nursing initiatives.

This appendix is not current and is of historical significance only.

- Secures organizational resources to ensure a work environment conducive to completing the identified plan and outcomes.

- Develops evaluation methods to measure safety and effectiveness for interventions and outcomes.

- Promotes activities that assist others, as appropriate, in becoming informed about costs, risks, and benefits of care or of the plan and solution.

This appendix is not current and is of historical significance only.

STANDARD 15. LEADERSHIP
The school nurse provides leadership in the professional practice setting and the profession.

Measurement Criteria:

The school nurse:

- Engages in teamwork as a team player and a team builder.
- Works to create and maintain healthy work environments in local, regional, national, or international communities.
- Displays the ability to define a clear vision, the associated goals, and a plan to implement and measure progress
- Demonstrates a commitment to continuous, lifelong learning for self and others.
- Teaches others to succeed by mentoring and other strategies.
- Exhibits creativity and flexibility through times of change.
- Demonstrates energy, excitement, and a passion for quality work.
- Willingly accepts mistakes by self and others, thereby creating a culture in which risk-taking is not only safe, but also expected.
- Inspires loyalty by valuing people as the most precious asset in an organization.
- Directs the coordination of care across settings and among care-givers, including oversight of licensed and unlicensed personnel in any assigned or delegated tasks as permitted by state nurse practice acts.
- Serves in key roles in the school and work settings by participating on committees, councils, and administrative teams.
- Promotes advancement of the profession through participation in professional school nursing and school health organizations.
- Demonstrates knowledge of the philosophy and mission of the school district, the nature of its curricular and extracurricular activities, and its programs and special services.*

---

*Adapted from Proctor, Lordi, and Zaiger 1993.

This appendix is not current and is of historical significance only.

- Demonstrates knowledge of the roles of other school professionals and adjunct personnel.*

- Coordinates roles and responsibilities of the adjunct school health personnel within the school team.*

Additional Measurement Criteria for the Advanced Practice Registered Nurse:

The advanced practice registered nurse:

- Works to influence decision-making bodies to improve client care.

- Provides direction to enhance the effectiveness of the healthcare team.

- Initiates and revises protocols or guidelines to reflect evidence-based practice, to reflect accepted changes in care management, or to address emerging problems.

- Promotes communication of information and advancement of the profession through writing, publishing, and presentations for professional or lay audiences.

- Designs innovations to effect change in practice and improve health outcomes.

Additional Measurement Criteria for the Nursing Role Specialty:

The school nurse in a nursing role specialty:

- Works to influence decision-making bodies to improve client care, health services, and policies.

- Promotes communication of information and advancement of the profession through writing, publishing, and presentations for professional or lay audiences.

- Designs innovations to effect change in practice and outcomes.

- Provides direction to enhance the effectiveness of the multi-disciplinary or interdisciplinary team.

This appendix is not current and is of historical significance only.

Standard 16. Program Management
The school nurse manages school health services.

Measurement Criteria:

The school nurse:

- Manages school health services as appropriate to the nurse's education, position, and practice environment.*

- Conducts school health needs assessments to identify current health problems and identify the need for new programs.*

- Develops and implements needed health programs using a program planning process.*

- Demonstrates knowledge of existing school health programs and current health trends that may affect client care, the sources of funds for each, school policy related to each, and local, state, and federal laws governing each.*

- Develops and implements health policies and procedures in collaboration with the school administration, the board of health, and the board of education.*

- Evaluates ongoing health programs for outcomes and quality of care, and communicates findings to administrators and the board of education.*

- Orients, trains, documents competency, supervises, and evaluates health assistants, aides, and UAPs (unlicensed assistive personnel), as appropriate to the school setting.*

- Initiates changes throughout the healthcare delivery system, as appropriate, using the results of school health environmental needs assessments, analysis of evaluation data, and quality-of-care activities.*

- Participates in environmental safety and health activities (e.g., indoor air quality, injury surveillance and prevention).*

- Adopts and uses available technology appropriate to the work setting.*

---

*Adapted from Proctor, Lordi, and Zaiger 1993.

This appendix is not current and is of historical significance only.

GLOSSARY

Client. Recipient of (school) nursing practice (ANA 2004). The client can be a student, the student and family as a unit, the school population, or the school community (faculty and staff). The focus of care may shift from individual needs to the needs of a group.

Plan. A comprehensive outline of components of care to be delivered to attain expected outcomes (ANA 2004). This would include an individualized healthcare plan (IHP), an individualized education plan (IEP) as part of the special education regulations (IDEA), a 504 plan, and others.

Role specialty. A practice in which the school nurse primarily works in education, case management, health education, prevention (such as adolescent pregnancy and parenting, or infectious disease), program implementation (such as special education or 504 plan creation and implementation), disease specialization (such as diabetes, asthma, or cystic fibrosis), administration, or leadership (such as lead nurse or co-ordinator for a large school district). This practice requires advanced study at the master's or doctoral level and considerable expertise.

School community. All those who study and work in a school district. This could be expanded when appropriate to community agencies, faith-based groups, student families, and others.

This appendix is not current and is of historical significance only.

REFERENCES

American Nurses Association (ANA). 1983. Standards for professional nursing education. Kansas City, MO: ANA.

———. 2001. *Code of ethics for nurses with interpretive statements.* Washington, DC: American Nurses Publishing.

———. 2003. *Nursing's social policy statement.* 2nd Edition. Washington, DC: Nursebooks.org.

———. 2003. *Scope and standards for nurse administrators.* 2nd Edition. Washington, DC: Nursebooks.org.

———. 2004. *Nursing: Scope and standards of practice.* Washington, DC: Nursebooks.org.

Marx, E., S. Wooley, and D. Northrup, eds. 1998. *Health is academic: A guide to coordinated school health programs.* New York: Teacher's College Press.

National Association of School Nurses (NASN). 1999a. *Code of ethics with interpretive statements for school nurses.* Scarborough, ME: NASN.

———. 1999b. Definition of school nursing. Adopted at Board of Directors Meeting, June, Providence, RI.

——— and American Nurses Association (ANA). 2001. *Scope and standards of professional school nursing practice.* Washington, DC: American Nurses Publishing.

———. 2002. *Issue brief: School health nursing services role in health care.* Scarborough, ME: NASN.

———. 2003. *Position statement: Role of advanced nurse practitioner in the school setting.* Scarborough, ME: NASN.

This appendix is not current and is of historical significance only.

Proctor, S.T. 1990. *Guidelines for a model school nurse services program.* Scarborough, ME: NASN.

Proctor, S.T., S.L. Lordi, and D.S. Zaiger. 1993. *School nursing practice: Roles and standards.* Scarborough, ME: NASN.

Synder, A. (ed.). 1991. *Implementation guide for the standards of school nursing practice.* Kent, OH: American School Health Association.

U.S. Department of Health and Human Services (USDHHS). 2000. *Healthy people 2010: Health objectives for the nation.* Washington, DC: USDHHS.

Wolfe, L. 2005. Roles of the school nurse. In *School nursing: A comprehensive text,* ed. J. Selekman. Philadelphia: F.A. Davis.

Index

Entries with [2005] indicate an entry from *School Nursing: Scope and Standards of Practice* (2005), reproduced in Appendix B. That information is not current but included for historical value only.

504 Accommodation Plans, 22, 60

A

Abilities in school nursing practice, 16, 73. *See also* Knowledge, skills, abilities, and judgment.

Accountability in school nursing practice. *See also* Delegation.
autonomy, ethics and, 27
for competence, 14
competencies involving, 56, 60, 65
professional, 13, 14

Activities in school nursing practice, 5, 13, 23
delegation and, 74
multidisciplinary (collaborative), 67
quality improvement, 56–57
quality-of-care, 71

Advanced Practice Registered Nurses (APRNs). *See also* Nursing role specialty.

assessment competencies, 33
 measurement criteria [2005], 113
collaboration competencies, 63
 measurement criteria [2005], 133
collegiality measurement criteria [2005], 131
communication competencies, 59
consultation competencies, 46
 measurement criteria [2005], 123
coordination of care competencies, 43
 measurement criteria [2005], 120
defined, 73
diagnosis competencies, 35
 measurement criteria [2005], 114
education competencies, 53
 measurement criteria [2005], 129
environmental health competencies, 69
ethics competencies, 51
 measurement criteria [2005], 134
evaluation competencies, 49
 measurement criteria [2005], 125
evidence-based practice and research competencies, 54–55

Basco, Delores, 86

Body of knowledge in school nursing practice. *See* Evidence-based practice and research; Knowledge, skills, abilities, and judgment

Bradley, Beverly, 88

Bryan, Doris, 86

BSN (Bachelor of Science in Nursing), 17

Budgetary issues. *See* Cost and economic control

Bulechek, G., 25–26

Butcher, H., 25–26

C

Care recipients. *See* Healthcare consumers

Care standards. *See* Standards of Practice for School Nursing

Care and caring in school nursing practice, 7, 26–27
competence and standards, 12

Case management. *See* Coordination of care

Caseloads and ratios in school nursing practice, 9–10, 28
[2005], 110

Center for Nursing Classification and Effectiveness, 25

Certification and credentialing in school nursing practice
competencies involving, 52, 57
numbers of, 18
as requirement, 17

Certified Diabetes Educators, 18

Chayer, Mary Ella, 86

Clients. *See also* Healthcare consumers.
defined [2005], 143

Code of Ethics for Nurses with Interpretive Statements (ANA), 1

Code of Ethics with Interpretive Statements for the School Nurse (NASN), 1, 15, 27

Collaboration in school nursing practice. *See also* Communication; Interprofessional health care.
[2005], 103, 133
competencies for, 62–63
competencies involving, 33, 40, 41, 48, 54, 71
standard of professional performance for, 14, 62–63

Collegiality in school nursing practice. *See also* Collaboration; Interprofessional health care; Peer/colleague relations and review.
standard of professional performance for [2005], 103, 131–132

Committee on School Nursing Policies and Practices, 6

Communication in school nursing practice. *See also* Collaboration.
competencies for, 58–59
competencies involving, 32, 40, 41, 43, 46, 60, 62, 63
standard of professional performance for, 13, 58–59

Communities in school nursing practice, 3, 7, 15, 16, 17, 19, 20, 21, 23, 25, 26. *See also* School communities.
assessment and, 33
collaboration and, 62
communities as healthcare consumers, 20, 7
community assessment, 18, 33
coordination of care and, 43
environmental health and, 68
ethics and, 50, 51
implementation and, 40, 41
program management and, 70, 71
resource utilization and, 67

Community assessment in school nursing practice, 18, 33

Community health nursing in school nursing practice, 20, 26, 63. *See also* Public health.

Individualized practice, tenet, 7–8

Individuals with Disabilities Education Act, 27–28

Informal learning, defined, 16, 75

Institute of Medicine (IOM) report on work environments, 8

Interprofessional health care in school nursing practice. *See also* Coordination of care.
    defined, 75
    as key role, 20
    in planning, 39
    quality of practice and, 56

Interventions in school nursing practice
    classification of, 25–26
    collaboration and, 21
    competencies involving, 33, 36, 39, 40, 41, 44, 47, 48, 66, 67
    mental health, 23
    purposes of, 8
    ratios and caseloads and, 9
    taxonomies for, 25–26

IOM (Institute of Medicine) report on work environments, 8

J

Journal of School Health, 87

Journal of School Nursing, 87

Judgment in school nursing practice. *See also* Knowledge, skills, abilities, and judgment
    caring as, 7
    as characteristics, 4
    defined, 16, 75
    professional development for, 17

K

Knowledge, skills, abilities, and judgment in school nursing practice. *See also* Critical thinking, analysis, and synthesis; Education of school nurses; Evidence-based practice and research.
    competencies involving, 32, 34, 39, 40, 41, 46, 47, 52–55, 61, 63, 68, 70
    as competency, 15
    education standard and, 52–53
    evidence-based practice and research standard and, 54–55
    knowledge defined, 16

L

Lamona, Eunice, 86

Language taxonomies in school nursing practice, 25

Laws, statutes, and regulations in school nursing practice
    Americans with Disabilities Act, 28
    assessment data and, 33
    competencies involving, 39, 47, 48, 58, 64
    delegation of care, 21, 74
    Do Not Resuscitate Orders in the School Setting, 28
    FERPA, 28
    HIPAA, 28
    Individuals with Disabilities Education Act, 27–28
    nursing standards as legal standard of care, 4, 31
    Rehabilitation Act of 1973, 22, 28
    student health and learning and, 26

Leadership in school nursing practice [2005], 103, 140–141
    competencies for, 60–61
    competencies involving, 39, 43, 56, 57, 63, 71
    graduate-level prepared school nurses and, 19
    role in, 26
    standard of professional performance for, 14, 60–61

Learning and learning experiences. *See also* Education of school nurses; Knowledge, skills, abilities, and judgment; Professional development; Student learning.
    competence and, 15–16